Getting to the
heart of
Cholesterol

THE HEART AND STROKE FOUNDATION OF CANADA

Yes !
I want to support The Heart and Stroke Foundation of Canada and its research and educational programs to reduce early disability and death caused by heart disease and stroke.

Enclosed is my cheque or money order payable to THE HEART AND STROKE FOUNDATION OF CANADA for:

☐ $10 ☐ $25 ☐ $50 ☐ $100 other $ _____

My name and mailing address are:

Name _____

Address _____

City _____ Postal Code _____

The Heart and Stroke Foundation of Canada is a registered charitable organization. Your support is appreciated, and a tax receipt will be sent to you.

Please check here if you would like to receive more information.

☐ Yes   ☐ No

Send to:

☞ **The Heart and Stroke Foundation of Canada**
1 Nicholas Street
Suite 1200
Ottawa, Ontario   K1N 7B7

Getting to the heart of
Cholesterol

CAUSES

MANAGEMENT

TREATMENTS

Dr. Howard S. Seiden

Department of Family and Community Medicine,
University of Toronto

Grosvenor House Press Inc.
Toronto~Montreal

The Publisher wishes to express its gratitude to **Merck Frosst** for an education grant which has helped to make the publication of this book possible.

Canadian Cataloguing in Publication Data

Seiden, Howard.
  Getting to the heart of cholesterol

Issued also in French under title: Le cholestérol : pour en avoir le coeur net.
ISBN 0-919959-40-7

1. Heart - Diseases - Diet therapy. 2. Heart - Diseases - Prevention.
3. Low-cholesterol diet.

RC684.D5S44 1989   616.1'20654   C89-093327-8

Published by

Grosvenor House Press Inc.
111 Queen Street East
Suite 456
Toronto, Ontario
M5C 1S2

Éditions Grosvenor Inc.
1456 rue Sherbrooke ouest
3ᵉ étage
Montréal, Québec
H3G 1K4

Cover design by Karen Paul
Printed and bound in Canada

The opinions expressed in this book are those of the author. Readers are advised to consult with a physician prior to acting on the basis of material contained herein. The author and Grosvenor House Press Inc. hereby disclaim any responsibility for any loss suffered by any person which results from a failure to so consult with a physician.

Contents

APPENDICES

About the Author

Howard Seiden, MD, MSc, CCFP, is director of the Front-Frederick Health Services in downtown Toronto, a preventive and educationally oriented, multi-disciplinary health facility. He is an assistant professor in the Department of Family and Community Medicine at the University of Toronto and has staff appointments at St. Michael's Hospital and Toronto General Hospital. He has served on the executive of the Toronto Academy of Medicine for a number of years and at present is vice-president. He was a member of the editorial advisory board of *Canadian Family Physician* and remains a contributor and reviewer. Well known for his medical writings, Dr. Seiden writes a syndicated weekly column that appears in many of Canada's major newspapers.

Introduction

Since its formation in the 1950s, the Canadian Heart Foundation's sole purpose has been the support of research and education aimed at reducing premature death and disability from heart disease and stroke. Throughout the years, what is now the Heart and Stroke Foundation of Canada has built its research support program from $3,000 in grants the first year to close to $28 million in 1988. It now sponsors more than 600 scientists and physicians conducting heart and stroke research in every major hospital and medical school in Canada.

We at the Foundation are justifiably proud of our contribution to the decrease in cardiovascular mortality, which is declining at the rate of two percentage points a year. In fact, we are now reaching the stage where cardiovascular disease can be prevented to a significant degree. Nevertheless, more Canadians die from heart disease and stroke than from any other cause, so there is still much to be done.

Nutritionists tell us "we are what we eat," and Canadians eat too much fat. It accounts for 40 per cent of the calories we consume, even though recent scientific consensus recommends it should constitute less than 30 per cent.

Elevated blood cholesterol levels put Canadians at excess risk of heart and circulatory disease. For many people a high-fat diet adds unnecessary cholesterol to the circulatory system. To help prevent this, the Foundation follows two basic strategies. First, it gives attention to high-risk groups by identifying successful therapies for high blood cholesterol levels. Second, it suggests modest lifestyle changes to the general public, such as reducing dietary fat intake.

We at the Foundation are particularly happy to be associated with the publication of this book because we believe it is important for Canadians to be aware of the risks involved in high cholesterol levels, and to understand how to maintain a heart-healthy diet. We hope this latest information on the causes and control of cholesterol will provide you with the basis for making responsible personal decisions about your health.

RAYMOND CREVIER   JOHN MCCREA
President   *Executive Director*

Heart and Stroke Foundation of Canada

Author's Acknowledgements

TO MATTHEW AND KERRI:

For regularly asking whether my book was finished yet; for having to spend their winter holiday without me because it wasn't finished; and for saying they missed me when they were away. I hope that part of the contribution I've made in this book will result in a better understanding of cholesterol, atherosclerosis and coronary artery disease and will help prevent the arteries of your children and mine from becoming affected. As a result of what I learned in writing this book, Kerri's and Matthew's diets will be more prudent.

And I thank Catherine, my wife, for her encouragement in the middle of the nights when I decided to call it quits and never finish the manuscript. And for reading the proofs until the wee hours of a work night.

Thanks to Isolde Prince and Kathleen Olsen, R.N., for searching, reviewing and charting the literature. And to my office staff, patients and clients for putting up with me. As well, I deeply appreciate the work of the experts who read and commented so positively on the contents.

For an author to admit that a book could not come to fruition without editors and publishers is a true compliment to these usually unrecognized yet vital people who specialize in reperfecting perfection. My gratitude to Fran MacDonald, Dr. Jo File and Julia Armstrong.

It is an honour to be the author of a book endorsed by the Heart and Stroke Foundation of Canada. It is not often that a non-cardiologist, non-lipidologist is given such an opportunity. I thank them for the privilege of this association and all that I have learned as a result of it.

HOWARD SEIDEN
March 1989

Publisher's Acknowledgements

The publisher thanks all those whose critical review of the manuscript helped make this book possible: Dr. Peter Olley, chairman of the Medical Advisory Board of the Heart and Stroke Foundation of Canada; Dr. Richard Lauzon, national director, programs, Heart and Stroke Foundation of Canada; Ruth McPherson, director of the Lipid Research Clinic, Royal Victoria Hospital, Montreal; and Denise Beatty, R.P.Dt.

PART I

Cholesterol

1

Introduction to Cholesterol

You're reading this book because you want to know more about cholesterol, its relationship to premature death from heart disease, and how the problem can be treated. Perhaps heart attacks run in your family and you've decided to look into ways to get yourself out of the running. Perhaps you're worried because a cholesterol test showed that your level is high. Or perhaps you're a perfectly healthy person who is simply interested in staying that way.

No matter what your reason, you bought this book to learn. We'll try our best to help you do that by giving you the following information:

- What cholesterol is and what it does in your body.
- How cholesterol can harm your arteries.
- The other risk factors for coronary artery disease.
- Therapies used in treating high cholesterol levels.
- Your own role in prevention and treatment.

But wanting to give information and deciding what information to give isn't easy with a subject as complex as cholesterol. The truth is, there is still much to be discovered about the function of cholesterol in causing heart disease. There is a lot more to be discovered about the effects of lowering cholesterol levels, particularly in women and children.

Those of us who have tried to keep up to date with recent developments in medicine are also aware that the experts in our profession have varying opinions. Recommendations change. Some of the research on which experts base their recommendations is not the greatest science. Medical studies disagree. Even special interest groups disagree. It will be our job, then, to present a balanced view of what the advocates and critics think.

You Will Decide

What you will find in this book is an examination of what lipids are (lipid being a fancy word for dietary and human body fat), how they're made and what our bodies do with them. You'll find information on the many other risk factors that can contribute to heart disease. You'll learn about therapies and which ones should be tried first. In most cases, the therapy first recommended is diet modification, so there are many pages devoted to nutrition and its components: vitamins, minerals, dietary fats, proteins and carbohydrates. There are shopping tips in these chapters, because the supermarket is often where the battle against cholesterol is lost.

Then you'll learn that your personality, your weight, how much you exercise, and the amount of stress you're under are also factors to consider. And since pills are far easier to swallow than major lifestyle changes, you'll learn when and if drug treatment is appropriate. There's even a review of major studies on cholesterol.

After sifting through all this information, you'll decide which parts of it you choose to follow and what advice you'll incorporate into your day-to-day life. You're not likely to follow recommendations that you don't understand. Changing a lifestyle without better than good evidence that it will make you live longer is something few people would undertake.

It's unlikely that any government will ever pass laws decreeing what you must put in your stomach. In the end, what you do will be your choice. It's you who will decide what foods to put on your table or order in a restaurant. And most important, perhaps, what food your children will put into their mouths.

By the time you've finished this book, you'll be able to recognize what's good for you: namely a prudent diet, exercise and relaxation. We may even have been able to convince you that what's good for you doesn't hurt. We can't guarantee that you will live any longer because of what's in this book, but you may.

Before we begin, however, you might be interested in some background on the discovery of cholesterol and its relationship to heart disease.

The History of Cholesterol

Cholesterol is far from new. In the early 1800s, the French chemist Michel Chevreul named a white, fatty substance isolated from gallstones "cholesterine," from the Greek *chole* (bile) and *stereos* (solid). In the mid-1800s another French chemist, M. Berthelot, replaced the "ine" ending with "ol" because the compound had been discovered to be an alcohol.

Although during the late 1800s there were suggestions that cholesterol affected the arteries, most historians seem to agree that the story should begin with Niolai Anitschkow's 1933 contention that cholesterol in the food we ate ended up as nasty deposits on our arteries.

Anitschkow's revelation came at just the right time. Coronary artery disease had been formally recognized for the first time in the 1929 edition of the *International Diseases and Cause of Death*. Prior to this, arteriosclerosis (hardening of the arteries) and heart attack (myocardial infarction) did not officially exist.

When the Second World War ended, giving medical researchers some time to study what had become an epidemic of coronary artery disease, one of the key investigators was Ancel Keys of the University of Minnesota School of Medicine. He looked at the death rates from heart disease of various countries and noted something quite startling: people living in countries with high incidences of heart disease had high percentages of fat in their diets. Keys also showed that feeding people diets rich in animal rather than vegetable fats increased their blood cholesterol levels.

A great number of discoveries about cholesterol have been made since, many of which you'll discover for yourself beginning in the next chapter. In fact, to date, 13 Nobel Prizes have been awarded for work connected with some aspect of cholesterol's obviously important role in our lives.

Cholesterol can be a matter of life or death. To keep you alive, your heart pumps blood through the coronary arteries, smaller arteries and veins to every part of your body. (The normal person weighing 70 kilograms has more than 100,000 kilometres of blood vessels.) Anything that slows down or stops that continual circulation of blood can cause a heart attack or stroke. Cholesterol contributes to atherosclerosis, which is one of the most serious obstructions we know, and heart disease and stroke are the major killers of Canadians.

A Few Words on Terminology

Coronary artery disease is a general term that covers many different conditions. Angina, for example, is pain in the chest caused when blood flow through the coronary arteries does not meet the demands required by the heart muscle. Arteriosclerosis is the term used for a group of diseases in which there is a thickening of the arterial walls; atherosclerosis is the form of arteriosclerosis in which the arteries are thickened and clogged by plaque formed from deposits of fat and cholesterol. Angina may be caused by arteriosclerotic narrowing or spasm of the coronary arteries. Attacks of angina are reversible, usually as a result of a drug like nitroglycerine. However, if the lack of circulation results in death to part of the heart, a heart attack or myocardial infarction occurs.

Another term you'll see a lot of is "blood cholesterol," used to distinguish the cholesterol detected in the body from that found in the diet. Some writers prefer the term serum cholesterol because, properly, serum is the liquid part of the blood. But we've decided that blood cholesterol is a fine description.

You'll notice, too, many references to LDL and HDL, which are cholesterol subgroups. As such, they are properly called LDL-cholesterol, or LDL-C, and HDL-cholesterol or HDL-C. However, there were so many references to them that our eyes began to cross. We have used the shortest term often, and even became informal enough to call them LDLs and HDLs. When the subject is as serious as cholesterol, you need all the informality you can get.

Summary

1. Heart disease and stroke kill more Canadians than anything else.

2. The higher your blood cholesterol the greater your chance of heart attack.

3. While we acknowledge the controversies and disagreements among experts in the field, and the poor scientific method associated with much of the research, enough evidence exists suggesting that certain lifestyle and dietary changes will lessen our chances of suffering from heart disease.

4. This book is intended to make you an informed consumer. It won't give you the right to practise medicine or nutrition science. And, even if it did, it is unethical and unwise to practise one's profession on yourself and family members. Only a foolish doctor has himself for a patient.

5. Take the information that you learn to your personal health care adviser to discuss how it can be individualized to assist you and your family.

2

The Lipids in Your Life

Lipids are fats and oils. They are a component of both our diets and our bodies. It is they that make food tasty; they that produce the enticing smell of pan-fried steak, fish and chips or fried chicken. Eating fats slows down the emptying time of the stomach, and that makes us feel full longer. On the other hand, even when we're not hungry, the flavours contained in the fat we eat may stimulate our appetites. Fats give food texture, as well.

Somehow, though, we've been primed to believe that lipids are bad for us - or at least that carbohydrates and proteins are more healthful. However, lipids in the proper quantity are invaluable to our bodies. We couldn't live without them. They form part of the cell walls, or membranes, that separate one cell from another. Vital chemicals, such as the steroid hormones, are part of the lipid family. Fatty substances surround some of our nerves, where they act like insulation covering an electric wire. Without this insulation, these nerves would short-circuit.

We get the fat-soluble vitamins A, D, E, and K by eating lipid-rich foods. Fat surrounds many of our vital organs and protects them from injury. The fat stored in our bodies can keep us alive during times of famine, which is one reason our ancestors evolved fat-storing cells in the first place.

When it comes to energy, lipids are very efficient. They store nine calories of energy per gram, more than double that supplied by carbohydrates or proteins. If we had to store our excess calories as carbohydrates or proteins, our bodies would be two-and-a-quarter times larger. Although there are lipids in all the cells of our bodies, reserves are stored mainly in our fat cells. And, as you may have noticed, they seem to have an almost unlimited capacity to enlarge with fat.

Triglycerides and Fatty Acids

It's easier to understand cholesterol if you're familiar with the terminology used to describe the different lipids. Most lipid in the body is in the form of triglycerides. And triglycerides are composed of smaller units called fatty acids.

There are three major types of fatty acids: saturated, mono-unsaturated and polyunsaturated. Saturated fatty acids (SFAs) tend to come from animal sources, such as meat, milk, cheese and butter. But some vegetable oils, such as coconut and palm oil, are also mainly saturated. Diets rich in saturated fatty acids tend to elevate our blood cholesterol.

Mono-unsaturated fatty acids (MUFAs) are found in olive and rapeseed oils, peanuts and avocados. The polyunsaturated fatty acids (PUFAs) are found in corn, sunflower and most other vegetable oils. Diets rich in mono- and polyunsaturated fats tend to keep blood cholesterol levels in the lower, more desirable ranges.

Until recently, the experts weren't sure whether to classify mono-unsaturates as good or bad fats. While it was once thought that they didn't affect blood cholesterol one way or another, researchers now believe MUFAs help to lower high levels. The evidence comes mainly from the data on coronary artery disease in such Mediterranean countries as Italy. The high amounts of olive oil eaten by the inhabitants of that part of the world seem to protect them from developing atherosclerosis. (The recommendations for how much of each type of fat we should eat will be found in Chapter 7 on dietary fats.)

Another short form you've likely come across is the P/S ratio, which represents the ratio of polyunsaturates to saturates in a food. It's calculated by dividing the number of grams of PUFA by the grams of SFA and is found on margarine and other labels. However, the major determinant of blood cholesterol concentrations is the absolute intake of saturated fatty acids, since they have a much greater cholesterol-raising effect than polyunsaturates have a cholesterol-lowering one.

How Fats are Classified

Most foods contain mixtures of fat, carbohydrate, protein, minerals, and vitamins. Right now, we're considering only fats, so let's look at the major components of three fats: butter, which has traces of protein and carbohydrate; and olive and corn oil, which are essentially pure oil.

All three of these fats contain SFA, PUFA and MUFA, but the quantities differ (see Table 2.1). To simplify things, we tend to classify lipids according to which fatty acids predominate. In this case, we'd call butter a saturated fat, olive oil a mono-unsaturate, and corn oil a polyunsaturate. The latter two contain no cholesterol, but you'll notice that the butter has 25 fewer calories than the same amount of oils. That's because a tablespoon of butter is 16 per cent water; the liquid oils are pure lipid.

Table 2.1 Components of Three Fatty Foods

One Tablespoon	Butter	Olive Oil	Corn Oil
SFA (g)	7.2	2.0	1.8
PUFA (g)	0.4	1.0	8.2
MUFA (g)	3.3	10.0	3.4
Total fat (g)	11.0	14.0	14.0
P:S ratio	0.06	0.5	4.6
Cholesterol (g)	0.032	0.0	0.0
Calories	100.0	125.0	125.0

Of the many different fatty acids, there are only two our bodies need but cannot produce from other fatty acids, proteins or carbohydrates. All the others we require we can make ourselves if they don't turn up in our diet. The two exceptions are the linoleic and linolenic acids. Since both are necessary for our good health, they are known as the two essential fatty acids.

These acids are essential for maintaining strength in our cell membranes. We need both of them to mix with other fatty acids, where among other things they help in the production of various hormone-like substances. Fortunately, these two acids are polyunsaturates readily found in plant and animal oils, and dietary deficiencies are rare.

Hydrogenated Fats

In nature, both MUFAs and PUFAs can be attacked by oxygen. When the attack is successful and oxygen bonds to the fatty acid, the food containing that acid becomes rancid or spoils. To retard oxygenation, the oil can be kept in a closed container and refrigerated. Another way of preventing spoilage is to add a natural anti-oxidant, such as vitamin E or vitamin C. Alternatively, a chemical anti-oxidant can be added to the oil. Examples are BHA (butylated hydroxyanisole) and BHT (Butylated hydroxytoluene), which you will find listed on many food labels. A third way to prevent oxygenation is to add hydrogen atoms to unsaturated oils, a process called hydrogenation. On the labels of foods that have undergone this process, you will read: "Contains [or may contain] hydrogenated vegetable oil(s)."

Why would anyone want to fiddle with nature this way? Well, aside from slowing down the spoilage process, hydrogenation changes the characteristics of the oil. Corn oil, for instance, is a liquid. But corn oil margarine is solid when it comes from the refrigerator, and even most of the soft margarines remain at least semi-solid at room temperatures.

When a vegetable oil is hydrogenated, it becomes more saturated. The proof is in its behaviour. Lard is solid at room temperature; chicken fat is semi-solid; corn oil is liquid. Of the three, the lard contains the most saturated fat, the corn oil the least. A hydrogenated corn oil takes on hydrogens and the hardness of a more saturated oil.

There's another potential problem with most of the hydrogenation processes. The end product has gone through a chemical change in which the fatty acids in the natural vegetable oil become trans-fatty acids. The catch is that with few exceptions, trans-fatty acids do not occur in nature. This means that most hydrogenation processes produce:

1. A vegetable oil that is less polyunsaturated and more saturated than usual.

2. Trans-fatty acids that do not have the beneficial effects of natural polyunsaturates.

The significance of our introducing these unnatural trans-fatty acids into our bodies isn't really understood. Some researchers claim we handle them more as saturated fatty acids than as unsaturated ones. It has been said that our cell membranes are able to make use of trans-fatty acids, but also that trans-fatty acids can alter normal cellular function. Other researchers have linked high doses of trans-fatty acids to cancer in small animals, although the effects of small amounts are unclear. Nothing has been proved, but none of the official bodies that have made recommendations on diet or cholesterol mention eating hydrogenated vegetable oils.

You may have a gut feeling that human beings simply weren't designed to eat synthetic food. You may be skeptical about processed anything and try to keep away from hydrogenated vegetable oils, including margarine. However, vegetable oils can be partially hydrogenated without creating trans-bonding. Although the process costs a bit more, there are a few such margarines on the market (see Chapter 7).

What About Peanut Butter?

If your children love peanut butter, you may be pleased because peanut oil is mainly mono-unsaturated. But most processors either partially hydrogenate the oil in their peanut butter or add hydrogenated oil to it. That way it lasts longer, is smoother and the oil doesn't separate from the solids. It also becomes more saturated.

Should you want no hydrogenation at all, at least one supermarket chain has a house-brand peanut butter that isn't hydrogenated and contains no additives. Or you could gradually introduce your family to the natural peanut butters that have no added fat, sugar or salt and aren't hydrogenated - they're simply ground peanuts. Many supermarkets now grind and package this type for their customers or, if you can afford the higher prices in health food stores, you can grind your own peanuts as you would coffee beans.

When you buy natural peanut butter, there's usually a layer of oil at the top. But it's not difficult to stir the oil in and little or no mixing is needed thereafter. Storing the container upside down helps, too. Lastly, since natural peanut butter contains no preservatives and may become rancid, it should be refrigerated unless you buy very small quantities.

What Happens to the Lipids We Eat

When you hear terms like "saturated," "poly-" and "mono-unsaturated," it is actually the fatty acids in a particular fat or oil that are being referred to. Now we're going to shift gears to find out what happens to lipids once we swallow them.

Under normal circumstances, we derive our fatty acids from food. And food rarely contains single, solitary, free-floating, fatty acids. In food, and for that matter in our bodies, most fatty acids are combined into the larger units called triglycerides. The triglycerides are a combination of three fatty acids and a glycerol, and they make up about 95 per cent of the lipids in our diets and our bodies.

Perhaps the best way to understand these and other very important players is to imagine yourself eating some fat. So picture a favourite dish - breaded pork straight from a Chinese restaurant, say, deep-fried in succulent beef fat. As you chew, the fats are mechanically pulverized by your teeth. If the delivery man was late and the food is cold, your saliva will be warming it up. A swallow and down the food goes, through your esophagus to the stomach.

Eventually, your stomach contents, fat included, pass into the small intestine. There the fat triggers the release of a gut hormone that causes the gall-bladder to contract. This releases bile, which acts much like a dishwashing detergent to emulsify the fat. The pancreas also comes into the picture and secretes lipases, which are fat-dissolving enzymes.

Now we're cooking! The triglycerides are broken down into fatty acids and glycerol. Glycerol and the smaller fatty acids are absorbed through the intestinal (gut) wall and re-synthesized into triglycerides. These are transported to the liver from the blood vessels surrounding the small intestine.

It's Not Over Yet

There are problems with the triglycerides. They don't dissolve in water and we wouldn't want them floating around in our bloodstream in the form of little globules. So in the wall of the intestine they are covered with a protein coating. The mixture of lipid coated with protein is called a lipoprotein. In particular, the lipoprotein formed in this way in the wall of the gut is called a chylomicron.

Being water-soluble, chylomicrons can float along in the bloodstream. However, they don't get into the blood directly; they pass from the intestine into the lymphatic circulation system and enter the blood from there. The bile salts that acted as digestant detergents eventually pass down to a more distant part of the bowel. They are absorbed separately through the gut wall into the bloodstream and transported to the liver. The liver picks them out of the blood and returns them to the gall-bladder, where they remain until the next fatty meal is eaten. At that point the process begins all over again.

The actual amount of cholesterol absorbed from your food in this process depends on a number of factors. One of them is how much cholesterol there is in the food you're eating. Another is what other fats are present in your gut at the time. Not all of the cholesterol you eat is absorbed; the rest simply passes through and goes out with your stool. The triglycerides, on the other hand, are high-energy nutrients and almost fully absorbed. Cholesterol isn't essential, and since it can be synthesized quite easily by the liver it doesn't require an elaborate, efficient, absorption system.

The Lipoproteins

We left our first lipoprotein, the chylomicron, floating through the blood. Most of the lipid in it is delivered to body cells with the help of the lipase enzyme. The chylomicron remnant is then delivered to the liver. As the body's fat-processing centre, the liver helps clear the bloodstream of fatty acids and reprocesses them for future use.

There are three other lipoproteins that make the news far more frequently than the lowly chylomicron: the very-low-density lipoprotein; the low-density lipoprotein that has come to be called "bad"; and the high-density one now known as the "good" lipoprotein.

Made by the liver, the very-low-density lipoprotein (VLDL) transports mainly triglycerides and lesser amounts of cholesterol to other parts of the body. Diabetes, obesity and alcohol may increase the amounts of VLDL the liver produces.

The low-density lipoprotein (LDL) is mostly derived from VLDL molecules made in the liver, and it transports cholesterol to other cells. A high level of LDL means a high level of total cholesterol. It is also one of the most atherogenic (causing arteriosclerosis) molecules circulating in the body.

High-density lipoprotein (HDL) is in the forefront these days because it protects our blood vessels from arteriosclerosis. It's formed by the liver and gut and, in a sense, has the opposite function to LDL. It picks up some of the cholesterol LDL has deposited in our arteries. HDL is also thought to carry cholesterol to such organs as the adrenal glands, ovaries and testes, where it is turned into good things like sex hormones and other steroids.

When you go to a doctor to have your blood lipids checked, a "full screen" is composed of:

1. Total cholesterol;
2. Low-density lipoprotein cholesterol (LDL-C);
3. High-density lipoprotein cholesterol (HDL-C);
4. Triglycerides;
5. Ratio of total cholesterol to HDL.

While some physicians still believe a test for total cholesterol is all that's required, you will learn in the next chapter why in many cases it is no longer enough.

And if you haven't already, you undoubtedly will be reading or hearing about other lipoproteins, such as IDL, HDL_2 and HDL_3, as well as apolipoproteins like Apo-A-I or Apo-A-II, B. Some of these lipoproteins may prove to be far more sensitive markers for diagnosing who is and who isn't at risk of developing coronary artery disease. Right now, however, they are mainly research tools.

Now let's consider the star itself: cholesterol. Found in all our cells, especially in the brain and spinal cord, it's also part of the bile that digests fats. It's the main constituent of gallstones and, as mentioned, the building block of sex hormones and other steroids. In the presence of sunlight, the skin uses a derivative of cholesterol to manufacture vitamin D.

If you consumed no cholesterol at all, however, your liver is capable of making a supply adequate for all your needs. It seems that cholesterol production by the liver is controlled to a large extent by the total amount of fat in your diet in general and, more specifically, by how much of the fat is saturated.

High levels of total cholesterol and LDL have been linked to coronary artery disease, including angina and heart attack.

Summary

1. Lipids are valuable components of both our bodies and our food. Most of the lipid in our bodies is in the form of triglycerides, which are made up of fatty acids.

2. Three major types of fatty acids are the saturated (SFA), polyunsaturated (PUFA) and mono-unsaturated (MUFA).
3. Diets rich in SFA tend to elevate blood cholesterol, while those high in PUFA and MUFA lower it to more desirable levels.
4. The lipoproteins are also important because a high level of low-density lipoprotein (LDL) means a high level of total cholesterol. But a high level of high-density lipoprotein (HDL) protects our blood vessels from arteriosclerosis.

3

Having Your Lipids Checked

Logic dictates that the first step in discovering your own cholesterol situation is to have a blood test. If all you want is a reading of your total cholesterol level, you need only present yourself to have a blood sample taken. The most simple test requires just a prick of your finger.

Some might argue that this is all that's necessary, considering the high costs of health care. Provided your result falls into the acceptable range for your age, everything should be fine. You have no need to be concerned about LDLs, HDLs or triglycerides. If your total cholesterol is normal, who cares about anything else?

The panel members of the 1988 Canadian Consensus Conference on Cholesterol had different views. In their opinion, total cholesterol, triglycerides and HDL cholesterol should all be measured (the LDL and ratio of total cholesterol to HDL are then calculated mathematically). But they recommended these tests as a priority only for those with a strong family history of heart disease, with known heart disease, or diagnosed as having diabetes, high blood pressure, kidney failure or obesity (30 per cent above ideal weight). As far as they were concerned, the country simply doesn't have the resources to completely screen everyone.

Another Canadian body, however, the Task Force on Periodic Health Examination, suggested that only men between 30 and 59 needed routine screening. That screening, in its opinion, should consist of a blood cholesterol test taken on at least two separate occasions, and a fasting lipoprotein analysis consisting of total cholesterol, LDL and HDL measurements.

On the other hand, the U.S. National Cholesterol Education Program has suggested screening every American over the age of 20.

The report of the Canadian Consensus Conference, then, has taken an in-between position on which of us should be tested, mainly because of the huge costs involved in screening every adult. Even so, if you are a health-conscious individual who wants to know as much as you can about your body, you may choose to ask for a full lipoprotein screen: total cholesterol, HDL and triglyceride tests. You may as well ask for the LDL and the ratio of total cholesterol to HDL cholesterol figures, besides. With all this information, you should know where you stand.

The Trouble with "Normal"

You should be aware, however, that many testing laboratories develop their own set of values for "normal" ranges by analyzing the results of a large number of blood samples from the people the lab services. Labs call this a "population sampling," and to fix a "normal" range they usually exclude the top and bottom 5 per cent of the results. The 90 per cent that fall between the 5 per cent excluded as "abnormally high" and the 5 per cent considered "abnormally low" are taken to be normal.

When a lab uses a statistical range of test results to establish "normal" levels, the actual result or "value" of an individual blood test isn't important. All the doctor or patient needs to know is whether the value was within the normal range, too high or too low. Depending on which of these three categories the results fall into, the patient may be given more tests or simply reassurance that all is well.

The only problem is that if the same sort of analysis was done in another part of your city, in another province, or in another country, the "normal" values would likely be quite different. And even the original sample didn't take into consideration such variables as ethnic group, sex or socio-economic status.

Clearly, there are limitations to the usefulness of "normal" values based on statistical analyses. According to North American data from the Lipid Research Clinics, fully 25 per cent of men over 40 have cholesterol levels that put them at about twice the average population's risk of developing coronary artery disease. If statistical norms are used to interpret their test results, most of these men will walk away with the false notion that they're "normal." While statistically they are, from the *risk* point of view their chances of developing the disease are higher than other people's. If they knew the real story, they might be able to cut their risk of dying of a heart attack in half by lowering their cholesterol levels over a period of years.

When Is a Cholestorol Level Unacceptable?

One of the major results of the Canadian Consensus Conference on Cholesterol was the outlining of "acceptable," "increased risk" and "high risk" levels for adults of both sexes. These are summarized in Table 3.1. The Consensus panel also made treatment recommendations when the LDL, HDL and triglyceride levels fall into unacceptable ranges (see bottom of table). The abbreviation mmol/L stands for millimoles per litre; mg/dl for milligrams per decilitre.

The Consensus recommendations will give you some sense of where you fit into the picture. However, this brings us to another problem with cholesterol testing. To be valid, the test results should also be compared to the values used in major studies of cholesterol, rather than to your "statistical" neighbours among the laboratory's customers.

Table 3.1 Canadian Consensus Conference on Cholesterol (Levels in both men and women)

Age	Acceptable	Increased Risk	High Risk
30+	5.2 mmol/L (200 mg/dl) or less	5.2 - 6.2 mmol/L (200 - 240 mg/dl)[1] or more	6.2 mmol/L (240 mg/dl)
18-29	4.6 mmol/L (180 mg/dl) or less	4.6 - 5.7 mmol/L (180 - 220 mg/dl)[2] or more	5.7 mmol/L (220 mg/dl) or more

[1] Intensive treatment should be considered if LDL cholesterol is greater than 3.4 mmol/L (130 mg/dl), HDL less than 0.9 (35) or triglyceride above 2.3 (200).

[2] Intensive treatment should be considered if LDL is greater than 3.0 mmol/L (115 mg/dl), HDL less than 0.9 (35) or triglyceride above 2.3 (200).

You are also entitled to some assurance that the lab that ran your sample did it by one of the recognized standard methods. "Accuracy" is the term used to indicate how close to a true value a lab was able to bring its test results. In an Ontario survey, it was found that a sample that should have read 5.2 mmol/L had been given a value of between 5.0 and 5.4 by 66 per cent of the labs tested. However, 5 per cent of the labs would have sent back a reading of less than 4.6 or more than 5.7 mmol/L.

"Precision" is the term used to indicate how well a lab tests in relation to itself. Given the same sample on a number of occasions, does it find the same results? In one Ontario sampling, half the labs had a precision rate of 3.9 per cent or better. That means, of course, that the other half had less acceptable precision.

Canada is not alone in this problem; a U.S. study of 5,000 laboratories found that 47 per cent of them produced test results more than 5 per cent off the real cholesterol value. Of those, 16 per cent were 10 per cent off the mark (plus or minus) and 8 per cent - about 400 labs - were 15 per cent off.

Little wonder, then, that the Canadian Consensus panel recommended that laboratories testing for lipids be expanded to accommodate increased demand - and upgraded to ensure that the results are both accurate and precise.

There is little you can do about this at the moment, unless you're a social activist prepared to question labs closely about their accuracy and precision rates until you find one with each rate below 5 per cent or, better yet, below 3 per cent in combination. Our hard-earned tax dollars fund these laboratories, but it is the rare taxpayer who would even report a lab problem to his or her provincial ministry of health.

One way around the problem is to have two sets of tests done, about a month apart, so that the results can be averaged. If the two results are very different, your doctor may want to have the tests done yet again.

The Best Approach to Blood Tests

So that the tests will reflect your usual lipid status, you shouldn't alter your lifestyle in the days before having a blood sample. Eat as usual. Sleep your regular number of hours. Exercise as you always do. Don't be on a diet to lose (or gain) weight. Don't change your smoking habits.

However, you shouldn't exercise just before giving a blood sample, and you should have fasted overnight. (No fast is necessary if only total cholesterol is being measured.) While your consumption of alcohol shouldn't have changed, both it and coffee should be stopped when you began the 10- or 12-hour overnight fast. (You are allowed plain water only.) Discontinue any medication you're taking if your doctor so advises. Drugs may interfere with the truth about your lipid levels, but your physician is the one to determine that.

Try to sit and relax for 15 minutes before the test. Postpone it entirely if you're not feeling well for some reason. If you're squeamish about blood-letting, ask to lie down while the blood is being drawn from your arm. If you want to be a stickler about proper procedure, ask the technician to release the tourniquet once he or she has inserted the needle into your vein; it should be released when the blood begins to flow.

Many factors can affect your blood cholesterol and other lipoprotein readings - the time of day, a change in seasons, whether you're sitting, standing or stretched out while the sample is being taken, how long the tourniquet is on your arm and when it's released. At the best of times there may be a variation of 5 or 10 per cent from one day to the next.

But if the lab chosen for your test is a good one, chances of the results not being representative will be less than 5 per cent. So increase your results by 5 per cent (for example, 4.2 mmol/L x .05 = .21 + 4.2 = 4.41). If they still fall within the acceptable norm suggested by the Canadian Consensus Conference for those of your age, odds are that you can be confident you have a normal lipid profile. If you're the cautious type, add 10 per cent and make the same comparison.

How Often Should Tests Be Done?

Those with acceptable results should have their tests repeated at some point down the road. If you have no risk factors for coronary artery disease (see Chapter 4), every five years should be adequate. If you do have risk factors, especially a family history of heart disease, testing should be done more often.

If your values are above those suggested by the Consensus panel, you and your doctor will have to decide how often to repeat the tests. Usually the second test is done four weeks later. Don't be tempted to try manipulating your results by, say, going on a strict low-cholesterol diet in the meantime. In the end, you'll only be cheating yourself.

Testing Those Under 18

Many doctors feel that a full lipid profile should be done on anyone under 18 if there is or has been:

- a family history of coronary artery disease (for example, a heart attack under age 55 in a parent, grandparent, aunt, uncle, brother or sister);
- a family history of cholesterol or lipid problems;
- a personal history of atherosclerotic disease.

You and your doctor will have to decide on the basis of family history the age at which the first test should be done. Some young people have elevated blood cholesterols that are genetically linked; indeed, children with some very rare inherited disorders have died of heart attacks before they reached the age of 2.

Because tests are covered by provincial medicare plans, most doctors would err on the side of caution and order them. If there's a family history that suggests an inherited problem, you might want to consult a pediatrician who has a special knowledge of heart disease.

Determining "normal" cholesterol levels for children, especially young ones, is a problem. We don't truly know their cut-off point of "normal." Should the top 25 per cent of results be considered to fall outside the normal range, or only the top 10 or 5 per cent?

If there's no family history of heart disease, any age from 10 to 16 might be considered for a first test. We know that the earliest sign of atherosclerosis, the "fatty streak," is often found in infants and young children. One source says fatty streaks are seen in the aortas of some children by age 3 but don't become visible in the coronary arteries until they're about 10.

Most of us don't begin to form actual atherosclerotic plaques on these fatty streaks until we reach our 20s. Perhaps the production of sex hormones coincides with changes in the fatty streak that eventually lead to trouble, or perhaps the sex hormones affect lipid levels.

For all these reasons, it would seem reasonable to perform a single test on otherwise normal children with no strong family history of heart disease only after they've reached puberty.

Summary

1. A "full screen" of cholesterol tests is a priority for those who have diabetes, high blood pressure, obesity or kidney failure, and for those with known heart disease or a strong family history of the disease.
2. The Canadian Consensus Conference has recommended appropriate blood cholesterol levels for both men and women.
3. You should not change your habits prior to cholesterol testing.
4. The test should be repeated if your levels are above those recommended.
5. You and your doctor should decide when a family member under 18 needs to be tested.

4

Risk Factors for Coronary Artery Disease

In a world as complex as ours, it would be naive to think that isolated occurrences are solely responsible for either miracles or catastrophes. Things rarely work that way. Very little of what happens to us depends on a single, solitary event. Usually, for something good to occur, we have to be in the right place, at the right time, well-prepared - and have Lady Luck smiling over us.

When talking medicine, it's usually best to avoid using absolutes like "always" and "never." It's especially wise in the case of risk factors - the circumstances that can increase our chances of developing a particular disease.

Part of what medical writers use when rendering an opinion on such things is statistics that other people have gathered in scientific studies and surveys. Even if the planning and execution of these studies places them above criticism, the best result the numbers can provide is a database from which risk factors can be calculated. In other words, the statistics are probabilities, not guarantees. But they give us a better guide for action (depending on how they were derived) than simply guessing or consulting a crystal ball - unless, of course, you're a certified crystal ball reader.

There are very, very few "major" studies that someone hasn't criticized on one ground or another. Either the questions were asked wrongly or the study method had flaws. Sometimes the results were calculated incorrectly. Maybe the conclusions didn't follow from the actual findings. And when these criticisms came to the surface, a body of opinion would creep forth to counter them, and yet another group would support them. All of which would leave us non-statisticians and non-experts in research design in a quandary as to what we could or should conclude.

Bearing all this in mind, it makes perfect sense that predicting who will or who will not develop a particular disease can be tricky. Sure, sometimes we can be pretty certain. For example, if a man locks himself in a garage with all the doors and windows closed and a car motor running, there is an overwhelming probability that he will suffer from carbon monoxide poisoning.

Still, the car engine could stall. Or the vehicle could run out of gas. Or maybe someone walking by might decide to open the garage door. All of which proves that rarely, if ever, is any result a sure thing.

Cholesterol is Only One Risk Factor

From a practical viewpoint, if we're going to be honest with ourselves we'd best admit that nothing as complicated as atherosclerosis can be caused by one single thing. Those who have heart attacks, particularly before they reach 55, often have more contributing factors than just an elevated level of cholesterol or a lipid imbalance. And common sense tells us that risk-factor analysis, no matter how scientific, deals in probabilities not certainties. One person may be at extremely high risk for developing a particular disease, then die of something totally unrelated; another with virtually no risk factors may have a heart attack at a very early age.

With all this in mind, let's move beyond the undeniable risk of high blood cholesterol to the other known or suspected risk factors for atherosclerosis. They are:

- Tobacco smoking
- High blood pressure
- Family history of heart disease

- Diabetes
- Obesity
- Lack of physical activity
- Excessive intake of alcohol
- Being a member of the male sex
- Type A personality
- Stress

Of these additional risk factors, the most important are tobacco smoking, high blood pressure, family history and diabetes. Most of the risk factors on this list, however, are amenable to modification, as long as you *want* to modify them. Which means that for many people - perhaps for most - heart disease and significant atherosclerosis *can be prevented or delayed.*

Let's examine three of these known and suspected risk factors in detail.

Tobacco Smoking

Statistically speaking, each cigarette smoked costs 5.5 minutes of life. For many nicotine addicts, that works out to a lifespan cut short by 10 years. Some very respected researchers have suggested that cigarette smoking is responsible for 30 to 40 per cent of all deaths from coronary artery disease. But we don't need to gather statistics on that point - any cardiologist will tell you that most of the beds in cardiac intensive care units are occupied by smokers.

Tobacco smoke increases the stickiness of blood platelets, small blood cells that can stick together to form blood clots. In essence, then, tobacco smoke makes the blood more prone to form clots. And clots in arteries cause the tissues supplied by those arteries to crave oxygen. They can't get enough. That oxygen starvation causes pain, tissue damage and death. In more practical terms we call these things strokes and heart attacks.

Increasing the blood's "clottability" is just one way tobacco smoke causes heart attacks. The smoke increases the heart rate, raises the blood pressure, and makes the heart muscle more vulnerable to arrhythmias - abnormal heart beats.

All of us, from time to time, have transient or passing arrhythmias. They're often called "palpitations" or "missed beats." Health care professionals call the missed-beat type a PVC, or premature ventricular contraction. You feel it in your chest as a forceful beat of the heart that seems to grab or startle you. As "premature" indicates, the beat came a little early, before the next normal beat was due.

We tend to suffer from PVCs when we smoke, consume too much caffeine, are tired or overstressed, and for all sorts of other reasons. If your heart is otherwise normal, occasional PVCs aren't likely to cause you any harm. Other types of arrhythmias can be just as harmless. In fact, some people's hearts beat irregularly for decades without causing them any problems.

More Sudden Deaths

On the other hand, there are dangerous arrhythmias. Some can kill within minutes. Smokers are more susceptible to sudden death than non-smokers, and one suggested reason is harmful arrythmias triggered by increases in the heart rate, blood pressure and irritability of the heart muscle. All are caused by smoking.

Carbon monoxide poisoning may contribute to the heart's increased susceptibility to arrhythmia. One of the by-products of burning tobacco, carbon monoxide bonds to the hemoglobin in our blood when inhaled. Hemoglobin's normal function is to bind oxygen in the lungs, then release it to the rest of the body. Without oxygen, the cells in our bodies suffocate.

For some reason, hemoglobin binds carbon monoxide more easily than it does oxygen. When it becomes saturated, our cells suffocate because no oxygen can get through to them. Tobacco smokers don't inhale enough carbon monoxide to suffocate themselves, but a heart muscle starved of oxygen becomes more susceptible to life-threatening arrhythmias. And that might explain those sudden deaths.

If you're a woman on the birth control pill, you're at greater risk of suffering from such cardiovascular complications as heart attack and stroke if you're a tobacco smoker. The older you are and the more you smoke, the higher the risk you take on yourself.

Tobacco and Your Arteries

Smokers tend to have lower levels of protective HDL and higher levels of coronary heart disease-promoting LDL. Perhaps that's why they tend to have more coronary artery atherosclerosis than non-smokers.

The aorta is the main artery of the body. Running from the heart down toward the pelvis, it then divides into the two iliac arteries that go on to supply blood to the legs. Along the aorta, branch arteries go off to supply blood to the arms, liver, guts, kidneys and other organs. Tobacco smokers are much more prone to atherosclerosis of the aorta as it runs through the abdomen. As a result, they're more likely to suffer from an aortic aneurysm.

In an aneurysm, a weakened part of an arterial wall balloons out under pressure. There can be localized ballooning or the defect can spread up and down the artery, causing a large segment of its wall to balloon or rip. When a major artery such as the aorta bursts, it takes only seconds to bleed to death. When the tear isn't completely through the artery, death may not occur for hours, days, or even weeks.

When an acute aortic tear happens, it usually begins in a segment of the chest artery. Symptoms are sudden pain in the front or back of the chest, or in both places, possibly extending to the abdomen and hip. Emergency treatment consists of getting the blood pressure under control quickly and making a surgical repair.

Some abdominal aortic aneurysms are found when a doctor feels a pulsing mass in a patient's lower abdomen during a routine physical exam. But about 30 per cent are diagnosed when patients complain of mild or severe pain in the middle abdomen or lower body. A ruptured abdominal aneurysm usually causes sudden severe pain, with an expanding pulsing mass in the abdomen and flanks. If bleeding is rapid, death quickly follows. The only effective treatment is emergency surgery.

Problems in Other Arteries

The arteries farthest from the heart also seem to be highly susceptible to tobacco smoke, particularly those of the legs. Pain starts if atherosclerosis has narrowed the arteries so much that the leg muscles and other tissue are starving for oxygen and nutrients. In the early stages, the pain comes with exertion; over time, pain-free walking periods become shorter and shorter. Eventually, there may be pain even when the muscles are at rest. If circulation is severely affected, tissue may die and become gangrenous.

Buerger's disease is another condition related to smoking. In fact, most of those who have it are young male smokers. Buerger's causes inflammation and blood clotting in arteries and veins, especially in the hands, feet, fingers, and toes. If the disease progresses until the arteries that normally carry blood to those parts of the body are plugged by clots, the fingers and toes die for lack of blood. The disease may not progress if smoking is stopped, but many with Buerger's find it almost impossible to give up their tobacco habit. And so they end up with amputated fingers and toes. Some patients design mechanical devices to hold their cigarettes after their fingers have been amputated.

Tobacco's Effect on Others

Most of us know that tobacco also puts smokers at risk of disability and death from a host of other diseases, including chronic lung conditions and cancer of the lungs, mouth, voice box, gullet, bladder and pancreas. Not enough of us seem to know that smoking can seriously affect others, too.

About 85 per cent of the air contamination found in a smoke-filled room is "sidestream smoke" from the burning ends of cigarettes. In a poorly ventilated room, non-smokers can accumulate significant levels of carbon monoxide in their blood, levels so high that someone with angina may begin to have pain. Other common reactions are eye irritation, headache, nasal irritation and cough. Tobacco smoke aggravates both allergies and asthma, sometimes very badly.

If we don't care what we do to our adult companions, we might at least spare a thought for the young. Studies show that children whose parents smoke are likely to develop recurrent bronchitis, pneumonia and other respiratory illnesses related to smoke exposure. Wheezing, asthma - and hospital admissions - are more common in children of smokers. Pregnant women who smoke put their unborn infants at significant risk of smaller birth size, premature labour and birth. And because the carbon monoxide poisons the infant's hemoglobin just as it does the mother's, the newborn is more susceptible to all the consequences associated with transient lack of oxygen at birth.

Smokers with other major risk factors, such as elevated blood cholesterol, high blood pressure, diabetes or a family history of heart disease, greatly increase their chances of having a heart attack. Even if you have none of these, if you are a smoker and you want to live longer the first risk factor you should modify is your smoking. Give it up totally. Both your doctor and the Lung Association can help you save your own life.

High Blood Pressure

The medical profession calls high blood pressure "hypertension," but some non-medical people get confused by the word. They think about being "hyper" or being "tense." So we'll try to avoid it where we can.

Depending on what figures one chooses to represent the upper limit of "normal," somewhere between 10 and 20 per cent of the adult population has a blood pressure reading that puts them at high risk of heart attack, stroke, kidney disease and blindness. In fact, even men with blood pressures that are only in the high-normal range are at significantly greater risk of heart attack than men with lower pressures. So it is probably fair to say that as long as you can walk and talk, the lower your blood pressure is, the healthier it is (unless it reaches 0/0, of course).

Blood pressure is measured in terms of two numbers. The first and higher of the two is called the "systolic" measurement; the second and lower the "diastolic." The systolic represents the maximum pressure in your artery and is recorded when your heart contracts in a beat. In between beats, when your heart is relaxing, the pressure falls to the diastolic level. Blood pressure readings are reckoned in millimetres of mercury, or mm Hg for short.

When people talk about blood pressures, they use such expressions as, "His pressure is 120 over 80." To save time writing, doctors scribble "120/80." This simply means the systolic pressure measures 120 millimetres of mercury, the diastolic 80. And 120/80 is a pretty normal reading. Virtually no one has a pressure of 122/78 or 118/82 because doctors, nurses and others trained to take blood pressures have a tendency to round off the measurements to fives or zeros.

What the Numbers Mean

In defining "normal," using real, not rounded numbers, we'll start with the diastolic pressures. Less than 85 is normal. Less than 80 is better than normal. That's something you should strive for. Between 85 and 89 puts you in the high-normal range. While you're still at higher risk than someone whose pressure is less than 80, no doctor is likely to prescribe drugs for you. At this point, it's up to you to pay heed to your diet and other lifestyle modifications.

A diastolic reading between 90 and 104 puts you into the mild hypertension category. Some doctors will prescribe medications at this point, others won't. It all depends on your other risk factors, and whether your physician subscribes to the theory that prescribing drugs for people with mild hypertension saves lives. If you fall in this range, you might bear in mind that in one large study, 58.4 per cent of the total excess in deaths associated with high blood pressure occurred in those with diastolic pressures between 90 and 104.

Moderately high blood pressure is defined as a diastolic reading between 105 and 114. If your pressures are consistently in this range, there's no question you have a problem that requires some form of intervention. And if your pressures run above 115 diastolic, treatment should be intensive.

Turning to the systolic pressure, you're allowed a reading of up to 140 if your diastolic is below 90. And so, while 120/80 is great, most doctors will accept 140/90 before turning to their prescription pads. Anyone with a systolic pressure between 140 and 159 is said to have borderline systolic high blood pressure. If yours is above 160, you're out of the borderline and into the actual systolic hypertension classification.

How Often Should Your Pressure Be Checked?

Every adult should have periodic blood pressure checks, at least once a year for even healthy people. It takes only a few seconds. If you have a strong family history of hypertension or your pressure has been borderline normal, you might want to have it checked more often. How often is something to discuss with your doctor.

Most people with elevated pressures have no symptoms at all. While headaches, ringing in the ears, lightheadedness and other symptoms occur just as often in those with normal blood pressures, the mythology about their being symptoms of high blood pressure may be a good thing. Many a patient with one of these symptoms has insisted that his or her blood pressure be checked, and at least some of those times a previously undiagnosed problem has been picked up.

As for the association between nosebleeds and high blood pressure, the medical books say there isn't one. However, anyone with a nosebleed serious enough to prompt a visit to an emergency department is usually pretty anxious and will tend to have at least a borderline elevated blood pressure. But the nosebleed causes the elevated pressure, not vice versa, and more often than not the reading returns to normal once the bleed is controlled and the patient is given a few minutes to relax.

Relaxation is very important when it comes to blood pressure readings. More than a few people's pressures go up just because there's a doctor or nurse in the room. It's called the "white coat syndrome." So if your pressure is on the highish side, ask if you can sit and relax for five minutes before having the check repeated. And even if your pressure is still elevated (unless it's sky high), you should be brought back on at least two other occasions for re-checks. Only then - and only if the average of the readings is in the high zone - should a diagnosis of hypertension be made.

If You Do Have High Blood Pressure

First of all, your doctor will want to make sure you're one of the more than 90 per cent who have "essential" hypertension. It's called that because we used to think that as people got older, it was essential that their pressure go up to push the blood through hardened arteries. Nowadays we call the condition essential hypertension when no apparent cause exists.

When there is an apparent cause, you'll be classified as having "secondary" hypertension. The cause could be various forms of kidney disease, gland or hormonal problems, neurological disease, or such drugs as the birth control pill. Your doctor will usually rule these out by asking you a few questions, and by ordering some blood and urine tests. He or she may also want a chest X-ray and an electrocardiograph to see whether the elevated blood pressure has caused any obvious heart-related problems.

In the majority who have essential hypertension, being overweight, eating a lot of sodium salt, drinking too much alcohol (more than two drinks per day), and suffering from stress may contribute to or aggravate the condition.

A diagnosis of hypertension should be taken seriously, but with the knowledge that it is only the very rare person whose blood pressure cannot be returned to the normal range. As long as you're willing to follow medical advice, high blood pressure can be treated effectively.

Unfortunately, many patients don't listen to medical advice. And many health care professionals have trouble communicating the very real need for their patients to get their blood pressures back to normal. As a result, up to half of those who know they have high blood pressure don't do anything about it.

Many patients don't want to take drugs, saying they'd rather lose weight, cut back on their salt intake and start exercising instead. Although this will certainly help and taking a pill is less desirable, the pill is easier. While these patients are working on their new habits, they'll have their pressures checked regularly (they can even check their own at home) and, as the lifestyle modifications begin to work, the medications can be tapered off - under the doctor's direction, of course. This way, it's possible to get their pressures back to normal much more quickly.

Another group of patients really has no interest in changing how they live. Most will accept medication if they are given some positive reinforcement along with it - and an awareness of how beneficial lifestyle changes can be.

The Care You Should Receive

Whatever group you fall into, a doctor, nurse or pharmacist should take some time to explain how your medication works, its potential side effects, how they and your progress will be monitored, and what's expected of you in lifestyle or other changes. (Impotence is one possible side effect and should send men to their doctors asking for an immediate change of medication.)

If you're simply given pills and rarely brought in for blood pressure checks and other monitoring like periodic blood testing, the care you're receiving is far from ideal. Some medications, such as diuretics (water pills), can be dangerous if prescriptions are simply repeated month after month. Almost all hypertension drugs have the potential to change the results of one or more blood tests. Without follow-ups, you'll really have no idea what the pills are doing to you.

Like everyone with major risk factors for coronary artery disease, those with high blood pressure must know their blood cholesterol levels. Having hypertension and a high cholesterol is worse than having either condition by itself. Add smoking and other risk factors and the odds of premature death are enormous.

Some of the diuretics, beta-blockers and other drugs used to treat high blood pressure can cause *elevations* of blood cholesterol. But some of the non-drug treatments for high cholesterol can lower blood pressure - dieting down to your ideal weight, getting regular exercise, eating a high-fibre diet, and lowering alcohol consumption, for example.

For more complete information on high blood pressure, consult the health or medicine section of a bookstore or library for a good book on the subject. Or write to the Heart and Stroke Foundation of Canada at 1 Nicholas Street, Suite 1200, Ottawa, Ont. K1N 7B7.

A Family History of Heart Disease

There's no question that those with relatives who've developed coronary artery disease are at higher risk of developing it themselves. Part of the connection is that other risk factors tend to run in families. These include high blood pressure, diabetes, elevated blood lipids, obesity, and susceptibility to tobacco smoke.

It's not universally true that nothing can be done about a family tendency to a disease. Some of what we inherit is just an increased risk rather than an actual disease or surething. If someone who's inherited the tendency to high blood cholesterol levels, say, happens to choose a vegetarian diet or live in a country where saturated fat intake is low, the predisposition may never develop into a problem. The same holds true for maturity-onset diabetes (see below). What most people inherit is a predisposition. If they maintain an ideal weight and eat properly, they may cheat their genes.

We can also inherit a susceptibility to high blood pressure caused by sodium salt. An amount of salt too low to affect others' blood pressures may cause ours to be significantly elevated. But avoiding sodium might well prevent this inherited predisposition from ever surfacing as high blood pressure or any of its complications.

Doctors generally become concerned about a patient's family history if relatives have had heart attacks before the age of 50. In most families no specific or clear-cut abnormality seems to link members who've had heart attacks, so it's likely the stricken relative inherited a number of heart attack-prone genes from several relatives. It's all these genes put together, along with such environmental factors as saturated fats and tobacco smoke, that caused the heart attack. This means that modifying *all* risk factors is important. There is no way of predicting which factor is most responsible for causing the heart disease.

Much less commonly, a single gene is the cause of heart attacks that run through a family. Numerous single-gene defects have been discovered, most of them involving elevated blood lipids.

Other Risk Factors

As mentioned earlier, diabetes is also a major risk factor for coronary artery disease. There are two types of diabetes. Type I generally occurs in younger people, does not tend to run in families, and invariably requires insulin treatment. Type II generally occurs in adults, particularly obese adults, and there is a tendency for it to run in families. While it can usually be treated with diet and drugs, insulin may be required in some cases.

Diabetics commonly have blood lipid disturbances. Because as a group they are much more susceptible to atherosclerosis, it is vital that their lipid problems be treated.

The symptoms of classical diabetes are increased thirst, increased appetite, increased urination, and weight loss. However, some Type II's have few symptoms and may actually be gaining weight. Overt diabetes can easily be detected in a routine urine test.

You will find rundowns on the remaining risk factors in upcoming chapters.

Summary

At times, it's very important to talk in terms of individuals rather than in generalities. If you're an average "healthy" person with multiple risk factors but no personal or strong family history of heart disease and you want to make the best possible lifestyle changes, here are some suggestions, in order of importance.

1. Quit smoking. More than anything else, tobacco increases your risk of premature disability and death simply because it contributes to so many different diseases.
2. Go on a prudent diet. Good evidence exists, and more is accumulating, to suggest that such a diet (see Chapter 6) will prevent not only atherosclerosis but some forms of cancer.

Suppose you've had your cholesterol checked and it's elevated, and you smoke, and your blood pressure is high. If your aim is to prevent coronary artery disease or simply go on living, your order of interventions should be:

1. Quitting smoking
2. Getting your blood pressure under control
3. Getting your cholesterol down

However, if stroke prevention is what you're concerned about, then getting your blood pressure down comes first, likely followed by reducing your cholesterol level then by quitting smoking.

The saintly approach would be to work on all three risk factors at once, of course. But lifestyle sinners may have to take them one at a time.

PART II

Treating Risk Factors

5

Introduction to Therapy

If you've been told that you have a lipid problem, there's no need to panic. No one requires emergency treatment for elevated cholesterol. But that's not to say you won't require therapy.

Most people with elevated blood lipids have "essential hyperlipidemia." You won't find this name in any textbook. The author of this book made it up, borrowing the term from "essential" hypertension. You'll recall doctors once thought that as people aged, it was essential for their blood pressures to become elevated to ensure an adequate blood flow through hardened and clogged arteries. We now know that the only thing essential about high blood pressure is the need to get it back into the normal range. And you may remember that "secondary" hypertension is due to some other factor or disease that we can identify and treat.

As with blood pressure, there has been a change in attitude on elevated blood lipids, a condition also known as hyperlipidemia. Even though studies suggesting a relationship between elevated cholesterol and coronary artery disease have been around for at least 30 years, it wasn't until recently that doctors paid much attention to hyperlipidemia. And even though there is reasonable data to support the relationship, many doctors continue to shake their heads when it comes to routinely ordering tests for blood lipids.

Also in common with blood pressure, the upper limits of what doctors accept as normal has fallen. It used to be that we called anyone with blood pressure or cholesterol higher than 95 per cent of his or her peers abnormal. We now know that the old statistical norms are inaccurate. For blood pressure, about 15 per cent of the population is at significantly higher risk of heart attack, stroke or kidney disease. When it comes to cholesterol, the number rises to between 25 and 50 per cent of the adult population, depending on age and other factors.

Again like high blood pressure, some of those with high cholesterol levels simply have high levels, probably because they have inherited a predisposition for elevated lipids. Others, however, have conditions that are either causing or contributing to the problem. Sometimes if these can be brought under control, their cholesterol levels will return to normal. These people, then, have secondary hyperlipidemia.

In Table 5.1 you will find a list of some causes of secondary hyperlipidemia. Because hyperlipidemia involves more than just high blood cholesterol, the secondary causes of high blood triglycerides are also listed.

Table 5.1   Some Causes of Secondary Hyperlipidemia

Hypercholesterolemia (high blood cholesterol) may be caused by:

I.   *Diseases*

Diabetes
Hypothyroidism (too little thyroid hormone)
Nephrotic syndrome (a kidney problem)
Obstructive liver disease
Multiple myeloma or dysglobulinemia (a bone marrow and blood problem)
Obesity

II.   *Diet*

High fat intake
High cholesterol intake

III.   *Drugs*

Some beta-blockers (for hypertension, angina, etc.)

Diuretics (water pills)
Anabolic steroids (used by some athletes)
Progestational drugs (some birth control pills)

Hypertriglyceridemia (high blood triglycerides) may be caused by:

I. *Diseases*

Diabetes
Chronic kidney disease
Cushing's disease
Obesity

II. *Diet*

High fat intake
Excessive alcohol intake
Excessive sugar intake

III. *Drugs*

Some birth control pills
Estrogens
Pregnancy (the elevated hormones act as "drugs")
Corticosteroids
Beta-blockers
Diuretics

You'll note the two references to diet as causes. Experts tell us that the majority of North Americans have diets too high in total fat, saturated fat, cholesterol and sugar. It then makes sense that most of those with elevated lipids can with some dietary changes (and more exercise) lower their cholesterols and triglycerides to a level where they are no longer at higher risk of heart disease. Information on these lifestyle modifications will be found in upcoming chapters.

Those with such medical problems as hypothyroidism may see their cholesterols return to normal when the underlying disease is treated. Those taking any of the types of medications that might elevate cholesterol should have periodic blood tests. If their levels do go up, the medication may not be absolutely necessary or there may be other drugs that perform similar functions but don't elevate cholesterol. In most cases there should be no problem in switching from a beta-blocker that may elevate cholesterol to another that doesn't.

When Drug Treatment is Needed

Once all obvious causes are ruled out, there will be those who despite very strict diets still have dangerously high cholesterol and triglyceride levels. They may well require drug therapy. Others won't want to change their lifestyles, in particular what they eat, no matter what their doctors advise. Certainly, as physicians, we would be remiss were we not to offer them medications to lower cholesterol and triglycerides, especially if they are middle-aged with cholesterols above 6.2 mmol/L.

To suggest that drugs are appropriate only if lifestyle modifications are unsuccessful or blood cholesterol levels very high is illogical. Several studies have shown that for every 1 per cent reduction in blood cholesterol over a period of years, there is a 2 per cent reduction in atherosclerotic heart disease. It follows, then, that using any safe method available to lower cholesterol makes sense.

Do You Need Therapy?

Needless to say, before embarking on any type of therapy for elevated lipids, you require a firm diagnosis. This requires a minimum of three blood tests. If the first one was part of a general blood screening when you were not fasting, the next two should be done after an overnight fast. The fasting blood samples should be used to measure all of your blood lipids not just the cholesterol, to determine which type of hyperlipoproteinemia you have. Breaking up that word makes its meaning obvious: hyper = high; lipo refers to lipid or fat; protein carries lipids in the blood; emia = blood. Put it all together and you have high blood fats.

If you didn't have a full physical examination prior to the first blood test, you'll need one to rule out secondary causes of hyperlipoproteinemia. One of your blood samples also should be used to run tests for these. The medical history the doctor gets from you should include a detailed family history to determine if anyone else in your immediate family has a lipid problem or suffered from heart disease at an early age.

Once all the results are back and you've reviewed them with your doctor, you should understand exactly what your lipoprotein problem is. Do you have a problem with just cholesterol or is triglyceride also affected? What is your HDL? Is your LDL elevated?

Have all the secondary causes been ruled out?

Next, someone should review your eating habits. Ideally, that someone will be a professional nutritionist or dietitian. Unfortunately, that may not be possible; their availability depends on where you live and what your provincial government is willing to pay for. If you are willing to pay out of your own pocket, you'll increase the likelihood of finding someone competent in a reasonable amount of time.

You might also try local hospitals or the medical officer of health in your community. Both should employ professional dietitians. If there isn't one available, consider other health care professionals such as nurses and doctors - but only if they have a special interest in the subject.

Once found, your adviser should be prepared to explain the principles of diet therapy with you. There should be time to answer your questions. The adviser should be interested in your likes and dislikes because an attempt must be made to tailor any diet to your own particular tastes. That doesn't mean that you'll be able to eat everything you want. If you're overweight,you'll be put on a calorie-reduced diet.

To control a lipid problem, the American Heart Association recommends beginning with a diet containing 15 per cent of calories from protein, 55 per cent from carbohydrate and 30 per cent from fat; cholesterol limited to 300 mg per day and a polyunsaturate-saturate ratio of 1:1 (equal amounts of each).

If that diet doesn't work, the fat content is reduced to 25 per cent of caloric intake by increasing carbohydrates to 60 per cent. Dietary cholesterol can be reduced to 200 to 250 mg and the P/S ratio is maintained at 1:1. This is known as a Phase 2 diet.

Since aerobic exercise lowers total cholesterol and increases HDL, it's reasonable for your doctor to recommend a program that you will be able to follow. In most cases, it is only after an attempt at diet and exercise has failed that drug therapy should be initiated. You'll find further information on this type of therapy in Chapter 11.

Summary

1. *Establish the diagnosis.* What type of lipid problem do you have? Are there secondary causes?
2. *Diet.* Review your present diet. Begin Phase 1 diet. Progress to Phase 2 as necessary.

3. *Exercise.* Should be part of therapy for everyone.
4. *Drugs.* Unless your levels are very high, these should not be introduced until the combination of diet and exercise has failed to bring lipid levels back to normal.

6

Nutrition Basics

Pâté de foie gras on toast. Cream of asparagus soup. Tomato and lettuce salad with blue cheese dressing. Lobster Newberg. Buttered baby carrots. Baked potato with butter and sour cream. Two glasses of white wine. Cherry cheesecake. Coffee with cream and sugar. A snifter of brandy.

Add the right companion, candlelight, soft music, and savour for a few hours. When all's done, the final course might well be left to your imagination.

Gulped down by yourself over the course of minutes, in between turning the pages of the day's newspaper, the combination will surely lead to heartburn and perhaps worse.

Food is different things to different people. To the gourmet, food is sensuous, offering aroma, taste, texture and beauty. To the solitary gulper, it's only a means of filling the belly. To the depressed or overstressed eater, it's often a quick high.

Regardless of the personality or motivation of the eater, however, once past the tastebuds in the mouth, all the romance of food is gone. For, alas, the constellation of sensations that entered the mouth quickly becomes a foodstuff to be masticated, swallowed, acidified, squeezed, attacked by enzymes, treated with alkaline, mixed with bile detergent, and eventually broken down into many molecular components. As you can see from Table 6.1, something as simple as an egg becomes a fascinating complex of chemicals. Some elements will be absorbed into the body for processing and

Table 6.1   Nutritional Composition of a Whole Chicken Egg

Proximate		Minerals (mg)		Vitamins	
water	37.28 g	calcium	28	ascorbic acid	0 mg
food energy	79 cal	iron	1.04	thiamin	.044 mg
	330 kj	magnesium	65	riboflavin	.150 mg
protein	6.07 g	phosphate	90	niacin	.031 mg
total lipid		potassium	65	pantothenic	
(fat)	5.58 g	sodium	69	acid	.864 mg
carbohydrate	0.60 g	zinc	0.72	vitamin B6	.060 mg
fibre	0 g			folacin	32 mcg
ash	0.47 g			vitamin B12	.773 mcg
				vitamin A	78 RE

Lipids

Fatty Acids				Amino Acids (g)	
Saturated (g)					
4:0	-	Cholesterol	274 mg	tryptophan	0.097
6:0	-	Phytosterols	-	threonine	0.298
8:0	-			isoleucine	0.380
10:0	-			leucine	0.533
12:0	-			lysine	0.410
14:0	0.02			methionine	0.196
16:0	1.23			cystine	0.145
18:0	0.43			phenylalanine	0.343
Total	1.67			tyrosine	0.253
Mono-unsaturated (g)				valine	0.437
16:1	0.19			arginine	0.388
18:1	2.04			histidine	0.147
20:1	-			alanine	0.354
22:1	-			aspartic acid	0.602
Total	2.23			glutamic acid	0.773
Polyunsaturated (g)				glycine	0.202
18:2	0.62			proline	0.241
18:3	0.02			serine	0.461
18:4	-				
20:4	0.05				
20:5	-				
22:5	-				
22:6					
Total	0.72				

eventual elimination; others will be eliminated without ever being absorbed. In the end, they are all recycled to the water supply, air or soil of Mother Earth. Isn't it a shame how science can ruin a romantic moment?

Calories are Food Energy

Your body is entirely unsentimental. To your gastrointestinal tract, a meal is only as good as it is useful. Take the dinner just described, if you dare. To your practical gut, that constellation of sensations is fuel to be burned as energy, like the gas you put in your car. That particular dinner contained about 1,950 calories of food energy per person. That's just about an entire day's recommended total for a middle-aged woman of average height and weight. It amounts to about 70 per cent of the energy required to keep the average middle-aged man fueled for 24 hours. Not that people run out of fuel quite the way automobiles do.

When you think about it, that meal wasn't terrible from a food energy point of view. As long as our average woman didn't eat anything else that day, her caloric intake and energy expenditure would have been balanced. She would neither have lost nor gained any weight. Our male friend, on the other hand, could have downed another 750 calories to fulfil his energy requirements. Were this his only meal, he would have been short about a double hamburger with cheese for that day. Unlike a car, however, he would not have stopped running owing to a deficit of fuel. People are better designed and have energy reserves to borrow from during times of energy-intake deficit.

The wine and brandy in our dinner contributed almost 250 calories. The remaining 1,700 or so came from a combination of carbohydrate, fat and protein. This brings us to a fundamental concept. Calories provide us with food energy. Alcohol has calories, and so it is a source of energy. Those who would exclude it from discussions such as this are being unrealistic. In the real world, many adults consume alcohol, often far too much. Even some who claim they never touch the stuff may admit to putting vanilla extract in their tea. It's about 30 per cent alcohol by volume. Like it or not, alcohol does provide a variable amount of calories for quite a few people. Nutrients, of course, are another matter, and we'll get to them shortly.

How Many Calories in a Gram?

There are four calories in a gram of protein or carbohydrate, nine in a gram of fat, and seven in a gram of alcohol. Which means that if one is considering only energy, gram for gram fat has it over alcohol. And they are both better fuels by weight than protein or carbohydrate. In other words, by far the most efficient fuel by weight is fat, followed by alcohol, then by carbohydrate and protein. (If you're having trouble picturing a gram, one millilitre of water weighs one gram, and there are approximately 5 mL to a teaspoon.)

The bulk of the protein in our lavish feast was in the lobster. Most of the fat came from the blue cheese salad dressing and the cheesecake. The potato and the cheesecake were the two top sources of carbohydrate. Why weren't the coffee cream and the butter and sour cream on the vegetables major fat sources? Simple: our couple didn't eat a lot of them. Two teaspoons of butter contain eight grams of fat, a similar amount of 18 per cent coffee cream, two grams, and a tablespoon of sour cream, two grams.

It's important that you realize there is nothing intrinsically wrong with such high-fat foods as butter and cream. In small quantities and balanced with other foods, their effect may not be significant. But eaten in excessive quantities, they're not high-quality foods. While you may get lots of energy per gram, they're like alcohol in that they offer little else in the way of nutrition.

The Importance of Balance

Nutrients like the ones listed in Table 6.1 may be converted to energy, have the potential to become a "building block," or participate in the maintenance and repair of our bodies. We can produce some nutrients from others, yet there are others our bodies require and can't manufacture. Called "essential nutrients," these include most vitamins, minerals and essential fatty acids.

A malnourished person is one whose nutrient intake isn't balanced. Even if body weight is normal, a person may be eating too much or too little of some nutrients. Our fantastic meal contained too few, and in some cases too little of the nutrients we should try to get in a day. It gave our couple only minerals and trace elements such as calcium, iron, phosphorus and copper, as well as such vitamins as ascorbic acid (vitamin C) and vitamin A.

Had our middle-aged woman used up her whole day's calorie ration in this one meal, she'd have been deficient in some of the nutrients her body needs. And even if our middle-aged man added a double hamburger with cheese to his day's intake, he would still come out short nutritionally. In other words, there's more to food than calories. We need balance, too.

For starters, no one needs the wine and brandy, even though their non-alcoholic constituents contain trace nutrients. So let's consider the alcohol to be a wasted, although perhaps pleasurable, 237 calories. You might call them "empty calories." That leaves just over 1,750 calories derived from food. Protein is contributing about 12 per cent, carbohydrate 33 per cent, and fat 55 per cent.

And here we meet another problem: the ratios are wrong. The Canadian Consensus Conference on Cholesterol has recommended the following dietary guidelines for those with elevated blood cholesterol and lipids:

Protein	10-15% of total daily calories
Carbohydrates	55-60% of total daily calories
Fat	30% *or less* of total daily calories

Other experts have made specific recommendations for the general population: protein 12 per cent; carbohydrates 58 per cent; fat 30 per cent. On either basis, our meal is fine for protein, very low in carbohydrates and excessively high in fat. Unfortunately, too many meals in the western world are just like it. In fact, our protein intake is usually closer to 25 or 30 per cent.

How Much Cholesterol?

We can classify the meal even more precisely. For example, it contained 38 grams of saturated fat and 12 grams of unsaturated. The total cholesterol was 635 milligrams. The more we analyze things, the worse they look! It has been suggested that we try to cut down on saturated fats and increase our intake of the polyunsaturated ones. And men aren't supposed to average an intake of more than 300 mg of cholesterol per day. For women, some authorities suggest a maximum of 275 mg. So from a fat and cholesterol point of view, our romantic dinner is a disaster.

From a vitamin and mineral standpoint, were it to be the average woman's sole meal for the day, she would end up with deficiencies in calcium, iron, thiamine and riboflavin, just to mention a few nutrients. If this were simply an isolated, poorly balanced meal, she could make up the nutritional deficits the next day. But if she were to eat like this all the time, she might well need vitamin and mineral supplements, as well as medication to lower her blood cholesterol. Our average man would be in even worse cholesterol shape after he finished his double hamburger with cheese.

Believe it or not, we've just covered many of the basics in nutrition. A balanced diet is one that contains a number of different foods that complement one another, so that when your day's eating is done you've received an adequate amount of all the nutrients your body needs. Such a diet will give you the right number of energy-rich calories, the proper protein-carbohydrate-fat ratios on average, and all the necessary vitamins, minerals and trace elements you require. It is called a prudent diet.

The Nutrients Your Body Needs

Because your federal government cares about such things, Health and Welfare Canada has published *Recommended Nutrient Intake for Canadians*, a vast listing of the amounts of protein, vitamins and minerals we need each day. Divided by age, sex, weight and height, the RNI amounts are set by a panel of experts but are not meant to be taken literally. They're intended to be liberal enough that everyone who eats approximately what's recommended should be fine.

After all, it's likely that we differ in our requirements. We spend our time in different places and have different activity levels. Even snoring at night could be a factor because the water loss of a mouth breather during sleep will be different from that of a nose breather.

The RNI chart separates the vitamins into the fat- and water-soluble types. The fat-soluble ones, A, D, E and K, are stored in our bodies for a long time, so consuming too much of them may be dangerous. The water-soluble vitamins are quickly excreted.

The RNI listings are in the process of being revised and should be available by late 1989. However, the federal government also publishes a very useful 32-page guide called *Nutrient Value of Some Common Foods*. It contains rundowns on more than 700 Canadian foods (including calories, fats, cholesterol and fibre content) and is available for $2.95 through the Canadian Government Publishing Centre, Supply and Services Canada, Ottawa, Ont. K1A 0S9, or wherever government publications are sold.

Guidelines for a Balanced Diet

If you need a direction in which to point your eating habits, Canada's Food Guide is a good target to aim at. Featuring the four basic food groups, it gives you simple guidelines on how to get the essential nutrients your body needs each day.

Milk and milk products: 2 servings a day as beverage or ingredient (children aged 2-11 need 2-3 servings; adolescents and pregnant or nursing women, 3-4). One serving is:

> 1 cup (250 mL) 2%, skim or whole milk, buttermilk, reconstituted dry or evaporated milk
> 1 cup (250 mL) yogurt or cottage cheese
> 1-1/2 ounces (45 g) hard or process cheese

Meat and alternates: 2 servings a day. One serving is:

> 2-3 ounces (60-90 g) cooked lean meat, fish, poultry or liver
> 4 tbsp. (60 mL) peanut butter
> 1 cup (250 mL) cooked dried peas, beans or lentils
> 1/2 cup (125 mL) nuts or seeds
> 2 ounces (60 g) cheddar, process or cottage cheese
> 2 eggs

Fruits and vegetables: 4-5 servings a day, including at least two vegetables, one of which is yellow or green. One serving is:

> 1/2 cup (125 mL) cooked or raw vegetable or juice
> 1 medium-sized potato, carrot, tomato, peach, apple, banana or orange
> 1/2 cup (125 mL) raw or cooked fruit or juice

Breads and cereals: 3-5 servings a day. Whole grain products are recommended; enriched are acceptable. One serving is:

> 1 bread slice, muffin or roll
> 1/2-3/4 cup (125-175 mL) cooked rice or pasta
> 1/2-1 cup (125 250 mL) breakfast cereal

Six to eight cups of fluids each day (water, juice, milk, soup, decaffeinated tea or coffee, watery fruits) are also important.

You'll notice, however, that the Food Guide includes some

items that may not be the best possible choices for those watching their fat and cholesterol intake - for example, the two eggs as a substitute for a meat serving. This is where Appendix 2 will come in handy to show you which of the suggested servings are lowest in fat. Choosing dried peas, beans or lentils (low in fat *and* high in fibre), the leanest meats and skim milk cheeses will help you stay in control of your daily fat intake.

Of course, if you're larger, smaller or more or less active than the average person, you may have to adjust the suggested serving amounts to stay at your ideal weight. If you'd like more information, Health and Welfare also publishes *Canada's Food Guide Handbook* (56 pages, $3.95). It's available from the same sources as the nutrient book mentioned earlier.

Summary

1. If you don't balance your caloric intake with your energy expenditure, you will gain or lose weight.
2. The ratio of protein, carbohydrates and fat you eat should be in accordance with prudent dietary guidelines as recommended by experts.
3. You should also balance your food intake so that you get all the nutrients your body requires.

7

Dietary Fats

You may have learned a lot about the fats in your body from Chapter 2, but here we're going to concentrate on the fats you consume or overconsume every day. After all, how well you control that particular habit is likely to influence your lipid profile.

You will remember from the previous chapter on nutrition that the Canadian Consensus Conference panel recommended we hold our fat intake to 30 per cent of our daily calories - or less. In addition, it made a recommendation on the different types of fats we should eat. Of that 30 per cent:

- No more than 10 per cent of daily calories should be from saturated fat (SFA).
- At least 10 per cent should be from polyunsaturated fat (PUFA).
- At least 10 per cent should be from mono-unsaturated fat (MUFA).

Since fat is more often calculated in grams than calories, you'll find a conversion chart in Table 7.1. As an example, the average man aged 25-49 needs 2,700 calories a day, of which 810 calories should be derived from 90 grams of fat. But he should take care to divide that 90 grams into thirds: no more than 30 grams of SFA and at least 30 grams each of PUFA and MUFA. In other words, 30 grams equal 10 per cent of his calories.

Table 7.1 Calculating a Healthy Fat Intake

Age	Average Calorie Needs[1]	Maximum 30% Fat	One-Third (Approx.)[2]
Women			
19-24	2,100 day	70 grams	23 grams
25-49	1,900	63	21
50-74	1,800	60	20
Men			
19-24	3,000 day	100 grams	33 grams
25-49	2,700	90	30
50-74	2,300	76	25

[1]   If you know your actual calorie intake, simply calculate 30% of it, then divide by 9 (the number of calories in a gram of fat). For example, 1,500 calories x .30 = 450 / 9 = 50 grams fat.

[2]   Amount of either saturated, mono-unsaturated or polyunsaturated fat consumed = 10% of daily calories.

This does not mean that average man can never eat red meat again. There's nothing intrinsically wrong with red meat, or pork, lamb or fowl, for that matter. There's really no such thing as a "bad" food; there are simply foods we shouldn't eat in large quantities. About three ounces of broiled sirloin (88 grams) has 188 calories, nine grams of fat of which four are saturated, and 64 mg of cholesterol. (This is where the book *Nutrient Value of Some Common Foods*, mentioned in the previous chapter, comes in very handy.) Even if our man has six ounces of steak, he's still within his limit for the day - provided he watches what else he eats.

It just isn't practical to deny people the things they love. A diet that cuts out your favourite foods is probably never going to work, at least not for long. It's far more realistic for you to acknowledge that some of your favourites aren't among the healthiest choices available. As a result, you'll be more likely to limit the amounts you eat, depending on your cholesterol level and the state of your health in general. And if what you crave appears on your plate less frequently, you may appreciate it all the more.

Cholesterol aside for the moment, you'll recall that whether it's solid, cooked, liquid, SFA, MUFA or PUFA, all fat has nine calories per gram. That's more than double the four calories per gram that protein and carbohydrates give you. So for the sake of your waistline as well as your heart, we present the following rundown of fat-cutting strategies.

The Butter Trade-Off

Butter is 80 per cent milk fat by weight; the rest is water, milk solids and perhaps salt and colour. One tablespoon (15 mL) contains about 11 grams of fat, of which 7.2 grams or 65 per cent is saturated. The remainder is polyunsaturated, and there are also 31 mg of cholesterol present. A lot for a tablespoon to hold.

But let's be reasonable. The pat of butter you get in a restaurant is usually about a teaspoon (5 mL). It provides 34 calories, 22.5 of them saturated. If you're entitled to 2,000 calories a day and 200 of them can be from saturated fat, you still have 177.5 left after you have the pat of butter. You may even feel you can afford a second pat.

Should pangs of guilt overcome you, order unfried fish with no sauce as your main course. Or have skim milk with your cereal the next morning. A cup has only 0.3 grams of saturated fat, versus the 5.1 in whole milk. On cereal, you'll hardly notice the difference in taste.

You have just made a trade-off. Skim milk has lowered your SFA intake by 4.8 grams. And your two pats of butter contained 4.8 grams exactly.

Of course, we're rarely going to have charts, tables, calculators or computer programs at hand to tell us these things so precisely. It's impossible for us to continually monitor the constituents of everything we eat to the minutest detail. What we can do, however, is start thinking about where we can cut fat and make trade-offs. Eventually it will become second nature, a good habit we've acquired almost effortlessly.

But first we have to learn how to cut fat whenever possible. For one example, butter can be extended by whipping air into it or by adding other ingredients. Dissolve 1/4 cup of gelatin in 2 cups of skim milk warmed in the top of a double boiler; add a pound of softened butter and mix well. Then just remould a new "spread" that only butter addicts couldn't approve.

And when you think about it, butter simply isn't necessary in every traditional case: sandwiches don't need any if the filling is moist or you use mustard or low-fat mayonnaise on the bread; fried or scrambled eggs can sit on dry toast (which stays less soggy); toast alone can taste fine with just a topping of jam or honey. Lemon juice is a far better taste sensation on many vegetables, and you'll read about alternate toppings for others a little later.

In short, you may find that the small package of butter you keep in the refrigerator for special occasions lasts for a long time.

Margarine

The fact that margarine is a manufactured product that usually contains vegetable oils creates a problem. As described in Chapter 2, the oils must be at least partially hydrogenated to stay solid, creating unnatural trans-fatty acids. So choose your margarine carefully. Becel and Fleischmann's Sunflower and Light margarines have the highest polyunsaturate oil contents and contain no unnatural trans-fatty acids. Some of the hard or stick varieties of margarine are almost as fatty as butter, and hydrogenated besides.

Remember too that, like butter, margarine is at least 80 per cent fat. Even if it contains a "good" fat, it's not saving you any calories. Only the light, diet or calorie-reduced margarines can do that. They cut calories by 50 per cent because federal law restricts them to 40 per cent fat. However, you can't cook with them, and the taste may take some getting used to.

Cooking and Salad Dressing Fats

Cutting fats and oils in cooking is easier than you'd expect. In most cases it's possible to decrease the amount of butter, margarine or oil or eliminate it entirely. True, the food won't taste quite the same, but it can be just as appetizing.

Frying should be done in a good quality, non-stick fry pan. Use one of the spray oils or just wipe the pan with cooking oil rather than pouring in a larger quantity. Melting fat from a piece of meat to grease the pan is not a good idea.

Try stir-fry cooking in a traditional wok. These are available in sturdy steel or with non-stick coatings; the shape depends on whether you're cooking with electricity or gas. You'd be surprised how much food can be stir-fried with no oil at all. You can use soy sauce, consommé, sake or white wine instead, but watch the additions that are high in salt.

If you bake, try cutting down bit by bit on the fat in your recipes; often it can be replaced by other moist ingredients. A good cookbook directed at diabetics or heart patients will help you experiment.

It's wise to choose single-constituent vegetable oils for cooking and salads, and to stay away from fully hydrogenated ones when possible. Table 7.2 outlines what we have to choose from, in order of their polyunsaturate content. Keep in mind that regardless of the oil, a tablespoonful weighs about 14 grams and contains 126 calories. Contrast that with the low-fat liquids you can cook or dress salads with: soy sauce (9 calories per 15 mL), white wine (10), lemon juice (4) and consommé (1).

**Table 7.2 Types of Oils in Order
of Polyunsaturate Content**

Name of Oil	Percentage of PUFA	MUFA	SFA	Characteristics
Safflower	75	12	9	Flavour not stable in frying but can be mixed with cottonseed oil; some varieties have more MUFA than PUFA.
Sunflower	66	20	10	Light taste; PUFA can be 75-35% depending on source, with MUFA of 50% in latter case.
Corn	59	24	13	Heavier taste; characteristic odour and flavour.
Soybean	59	23	14	May have unpleasant smell or flavour when unhydrogenated or used for frying.
Cottonseed	52	18	26	Good general-purpose oil with strong, sometimes nut-like flavour.
Sesame	40	40	18	Strong taste but equal parts of PUFA and MUFA make it a good health choice.

Peanut	32	46	17	Strong taste; tends to solidify when refrigerated; unhydrogenated may be deodorized to give it a bland taste.
Canola	32	62	6	Good salad or cooking oil; made from rapeseed.
Olive	15	71	14	Excellent salad or cooking oil; highest in MUFA (see next section).
Palm	10	38	52	Producers claim MUFA content balances out high SFA; until better research available use caution when buying products that contain it.
Palm Kernel	2	10	80	SFA higher than butter; avoid.
Coconut	2	6	97	SFA far higher than butter; avoid.

More on Olive Oil

Because of recent claims suggesting that mono-unsaturates are particularly desirable in our diets, we'd best take a more detailed look at the oil that has more MUFA than any other.

Interest in the benefits of olive oil resulted from data indicating that Mediterranean people, particularly Italians and Greeks, have lower incidences of heart disease than Americans or Finns (who consume more saturated fats). In the early 1980s reports suggested that olive oil's mono-unsaturated fatty acids gave it anti-atherosclerotic properties.

If this raised your own interest in olive oil, you may have noticed that there are different grades in the supermarket, and thus different prices. The grades or qualities are set by the International Olive Oil Council, to which 96 per cent of the world's producers belong. The following listing of its classifications may help you decide.

- "Virgin" olive oil may be made only by mechanical or other physical methods, which normally means pressing the olives.
- "Extra" virgin olive oil has to be of absolutely perfect flavour and odour.
- "Fine" virgin must also have perfect flavour and odour but is slightly more acidic.

- "Semi-fine" or "Ordinary" virgin must have good flavour and odour and is again slightly more acidic.
- "Refined" olive oil is obtained by processing virgin olive oils. It has an acceptable odour and taste, and is light yellow compared to the virgin oil's light-yellow-to-green colour.
- "Olive oil" or "Pure olive oil" consists of a blend of virgin and refined oils. It has good odour and flavour and is light yellow to green.

All grades are probably equal from a nutritional point of view. The amino acid content varies depending on where and how the olives were grown, not on the grade. So which one you buy will depend on your taste buds, sense of smell, disposable income and snobbishness level. (It's rather like the difference between plain cognac, VS, VSOP and XO.) If you've never liked the taste or smell of olive oil, one of the more expensive types may change your mind.

Mayonnaise and Other Salad Dressings

The federal Food and Drug Act defines what constituents products must have to be called mayonnaise or salad dressing. Regular mayonnaise must contain at least 65 per cent oil; regular salad dressing at least 35 per cent vegetable oil.

Those of you who really want to control what you eat will find recipes for your own mayonnaises and dressings. You can cut down on oil by adding orange or apple juice, for example. Creamy dressings can be made with low-fat plain yogurt. Be creative enough and you may become renowned for your "house" dressing.

Milk and Cream

Whole or homogenized milk has 8 grams of fat per cup, 2 per cent milk has 5, and skim has virtually none at all. Buttermilk, a fermented milk product, has about 2 grams per cup; goat's milk, which some drink because they're convinced it's good for them, is very high-fat with 10 grams per cup.

If you're drinking whole milk, a change to skim may be too much for you all at once. Move to 2 per cent for a week or so, then try a 1 per cent mixture: equal parts of skim and 2 per cent. Think of whole milk as skim with two pats of butter in it and you may feel better about taking the final step.

None of us should be consuming large quantities of cream. But if you truly love that morning cup of coffee and it just doesn't taste the same without half-and-half, you may decide that the 20 calories and 2 grams of fat (1.1 saturated) in a tablespoonful are worth it. (One of those little coffee cream containers holds a little more - 20 mL vs the 15 mL in a tablespoon.)

Prejudice is prejudice even when it's aimed at food; cream isn't bad for you unless you consume a lot of it. Sugar isn't terrible either: 2 teaspoons add only 30 calories and no fat. If that wake-up coffee with these small amounts of cream and sugar is worth 50 calories to you, have it. But if you're drinking 10 cups a day, 500 calories and 20 grams of fat may cause problems, as may the overdose of caffeine you'll be getting.

As for non-dairy coffee whiteners, one look at the ingredient label and you'll see why some people call them inedible oil products. They often contain coconut oil, more highly saturated than butter. If there's nothing else available and you can't stand coffee black, maybe you should reconsider drinking coffee at all.

Cheese

Most cheeses are surprisingly high in both saturated fat and calories. If you're watching your intake of either, you'd better become a careful reader of labels to find the low-fat varieties. Labels list both moisture and fat contents; as Appendix 2 will tell you, just 1-1/2 ounces (45 g) of most hard cheeses have up to 15 grams of fat. And it is at least 60 per cent saturated.

The choice of low-fat and skim milk cheeses may get larger as consumers become more health-conscious. If you find such cheeses bland, liven them up with a sprinkling of pepper, curry powder or other spice. Or try a commercial herb-spice blend that doesn't contain salt. There are many of these on the market and you may find them invaluable in helping you get used to the new tastes of a low-fat diet.

Yogurt and Sour Cream

Plain yogurt gives you the nutritional content of the milk from which it was made, minus some of the lactate (milk sugar) that its lactobacillus bacteria ferment to lactic acid. Apparently these harmless bacteria can withstand the human digestive process, which means they'll be in the colon as long as yogurt is eaten regularly. This may be beneficial, since there is some evidence that populations consuming large amounts of yogurt have fewer cases of colon cancer. This has not been proven, however.

The many yogurts available differ in fat content, flavouring and sweetener content. Those watching both calories and fat will want to choose the ones with the lowest butterfat (B.F.) content and no added sugar or honey. The butterfat content of frozen fruit yogurt can be more than 6 per cent, but there are yogurts on the market with less than 1 per cent. As well, some are sweetened with non-nutritive sweeteners that add few or no calories.

Sour cream with a 14 per cent B.F. content has 2 grams of fat, 6 mg of cholesterol and 23 calories per tablespoon. There are "light" versions with half the fat and calories, but you can do even better with a plain yogurt that's very low in fat. Try it on baked or sweet potatoes or anywhere else you're tempted to use gobs of sour cream or butter. (Here too a sprinkling of pepper, herb or spice will help.) You may find it hard to believe at first, but there are some who now swear they'll never eat sour cream again.

Ice Cream

As you'll see in Appendix 2, regular ice creams have about 16 grams of fat per cup; specialty or gourmet brands may have 24. Soft-serve ice cream is one of the types that contains high quantities of fat, 22 g per cup. If you truly have to have ice cream, go for small quantities, occasionally. Three ounces of the plain type will furnish you with about 100 calories, 5 grams of fat (3.3 saturated) and 22 mg of cholesterol. You can afford that as long as you compensate with the rest of the food you eat that day - and have the willpower to stop after 3 ounces. There are low-fat, calorie-reduced "ice creams" on the market, or you can move into sorbets or sherbets. Tofutti is an ice cream substitute made with tofu (soy).

Eggs

The only difference between white and brown eggs is the color of the shell. All of an egg's cholesterol (272 mg) and fat (5 grams: 2 SFA; 2 MUFA; 1 PUFA) are in the yolk. If you've been advised to limit your daily cholesterol to 300 mg, then one single large egg has you well on your way. Egg yolks aren't something you should be consuming on a regular basis.

In some recipes, two egg whites can be substituted for one whole egg. Or you can use a teaspoon of cornstarch in place of an egg yolk to thicken sauces. You can also buy cholesterol-free egg substitutes.

Some experts feel that eggs have been over-rated as a source of nutrients, saying that although they contain some protein, their cholesterol content is higher than most other protein sources.

But if you like eggs and you've been advised to simply limit your saturated fats and calories, you may want to keep them as a regular part of your diet unless subsequent cholesterol tests indicate that they're causing problems. At least two studies,one American and one British, have shown that eggs do not cause everyone's cholesterol levels to increase. However, the levels in an estimated third of the population *will* go up if they eat foods high in cholesterol. And the only way to identify these "hyper-responders" is to test how they react to various diets.

Poultry

Choose chicken and turkey over goose and duck, and remove the skin before you cook them. That's because the fat in fowl lies under the skin. Eating it or frying your bird could double your fat intake. Broil it, or roast it on a rack so the fat can drain off. Rejoice if you prefer white meat; it's more lean than the dark. And think twice about gravy. Does tender, sweet chicken really need any?

Meats

In general, breeders have been producing animals with a greater proportion of lean to fat. But don't interpret that to mean all the butcher's cuts of meat are lean. Cuts from the leg are leaner, from the loin a little fatter, and from the shoulder, fatter still. Lean cuts of beef include round, sirloin, flank steak, tenderloin and chipped beef. Lean pork cuts include lean fresh ham, canned, cured or boiled ham, back bacon and tenderloin. All cuts of veal except for the cutlets are considered to be lean. Medium-fat meats include most other beef, pork and lamb cuts.

Trim any visible fat from meat before you cook it. You'll be surprised what a difference that alone can make. An untrimmed rib roast is 20 per cent fat, but that can be reduced to 11 per cent with a good trimming. A rump roast can be reduced from 11 per cent to 8. Organ meats such as liver and kidney are high in cholesterol: 3.5 ounces of beef liver has 440 mg; an equivalent amount of kidney, 700 mg.

While you may consider side bacon to be a meat, many nutritionists classify it with the fats because even when cooked crisp it has more fat than protein. The actual ratio is 3 to 2. Three slices (19 g) of bacon are about 109 calories and 9 grams of fat (3.3 SFA, 4.5 MUFA and 1.1 PUFA).

When preparing any meat, barbecue, steam, broil, bake, roast or microwave it rather than fry or deep fry. And cook it on a rack too so that the melting fat is given a chance to fall away.

If from time to time you'd like to avoid meat altogether, high-protein substitutes are available at health food stores. These include beef and chicken taste-alikes made with soy protein. You can dilute ground beef yourself by adding soyburger. (Of course, you bought lean ground beef to start with.)

When eating beef in a restaurant, order the filet. It's generally smaller than other steaks and its fat content is among the lowest. That's why filets tend to be cooked wrapped in bacon; if you're really serious about reducing fat, ask that yours be cooked without its wrapping.

Naturally, you're aware that such luncheon meats as bologna, salami, sausage, bratwurst, knackwurst, hot dogs, frankfurters and the like are all high in fat; some can be 40 per cent or more. According to manufacturers, it's possible to make low-fat hot dogs, sausages and cold cuts but the public won't buy them. At least the public never used to buy them. That may well change. There are now low-fat sandwich meats available either packaged or cut at the meat counter. Buy them and show your support.

Fish

Those who eat fish regularly are less likely to suffer from coronary artery disease than those who eat it occasionally or not at all. It has been suggested that this is due in part to omega-3 fatty acids, which are found in fatty fish such as salmon and mackerel.

The two omega-3 polyunsaturated fatty acids that have received attention are EPA (eicosapentaenoic acid) and DHA (docosahexaenoic acid). Someday fairly soon you can expect to see processed products containing them being promoted as healthy foods. A great deal of food industry research is being carried on, and a number of major companies already have patents. Quite properly, Canada does not allow omega-3 fatty acids to be sold as food supplements. In the U.S. they can be bought in capsule form in drug and health food stores. Our government has decided they are drugs, not food additives, which means that anyone who wants to market them will have to apply for a new drug licence. It's unlikely that any company will do the research needed to apply.

Cod liver supplements should *not* be used as omega-3 supplements. You'd have to take about 10 capsules per day and that could well lead to serious vitamin A and D poisoning.

If you can manage it, three to five fish meals per week would be great. Cod, halibut, sole, whitefish and bluefish have less fat and fewer calories than tuna, sardines, salmon and mackerel. The fish highest in omega-3 fatty acids are mackerel, sardines, salmon, whitefish, anchovies, sablefish and tuna. Fish moderately high include bass, bluefish, hake, halibut, mullet, ocean perch, pollock, rainbow trout, rockfish, sea trout and smelt.

Canned fish is often packed in oil. Check the labels and, if there's a choice, buy water-packed fish. When you must purchase oil-packed, drain the fish well - especially if you're watching calories.

Clams, oysters and scallops are lower in fat and cholesterol than other meats and seafoods. Shrimp, lobster and crab are reasonably high in cholesterol compared to other shellfish, but much lower than eggs or liver.

Fruits and Vegetables

With few exceptions, fruits and vegetables are fat-free. Unless, of course, you fry them in oil or sauté them in butter or drown them with a rich sauce. One exception to the fat-free rule is the avocado, about which you will learn more in Appendix 2. Its fat is mainly mono-unsaturated and few people devour avocados, but if you add mayonnaise you'll have a very fat-heavy treat.

You'll find more on fruits and vegetables in Chapter 9, where you'll also read about the possibility that some of them may affect cholesterol levels positively rather than negatively.

Nuts

There are varying amounts of saturated fat in nuts. On the lower end of the scale are walnuts, pecans, almonds, peanuts (which are actually legumes), hazelnuts and brazil nuts. All have 5-10 grams of saturated fat per cup. Higher are cashews and macadamia nuts with 13-15 grams per cup; highest is coconut with 45 grams. A tablespoon of processed peanut butter contains 1.5 grams of saturated fat (and probably some sugar and salt). Processed nuts are high in both fat and calories: 1/2 cup of oil-roasted peanuts provides 447 calories and 38 grams of fat.

Breads, Baked Goods, Cereals and Pastas

Breads, pita bread, tortillas and cereals made from whole grains contain only traces of fat, unless it has been added (check the label). You could bake bread yourself and so know exactly what's in it; if you can stand the price tag there are now automatic bread-making machines to which you just add the ingredients and set a timer. It's even possible to have the baking finish precisely at the time your alarm clock goes off in the morning!

Bakery goods such as doughnuts, croissants, cakes, pastries and cookies are usually high in fat. Try to choose lower-fat ones, like arrowroot cookies, or bake your own using less fat and oil. Crackers are surprisingly high in fat, often including hydrogenated oils and palm oil. Soda biscuits, melba toast, rice cakes and water biscuits have less fat than most.

Virtually every cereal you can think of has significantly fewer calories and fat than the granolas. Often made with palm or coconut oil and sugar, a half cup of granola contains about 17 grams of fat and 300 calories. A half-cup of oatmeal has 1 gram of fat and 70 calories.

Check the labels when buying any type of pasta. Some contain only trace amounts of fat from the grains they're made from; others have added fats or oils. Some pasta contains eggs. While pasta is increasingly available in bulk form, either fresh or dried, the stores that sell it this way rarely have any idea what's in it. Nor do restaurants know what's in the pasta they serve.

Desserts, Spreads and Candy

If you're not content with fresh fruit for dessert (with or without low-fat yogurt), try puddings made with skim milk, gelatin desserts, sorbet or tofutti. Avoid anything laced with sugar or covered with whipped cream.

Marmite is a yeast extract spread that takes some getting used to, but it is well worth the effort and very nutritious. Like jam, marmalade and honey, it is fat-free, although all contain sugar. Limit your intake of canned or packaged meat and fish pastes, which tend to have a lot of fat.

As for candy, try to avoid toffee, fudge and butterscotch made with butter. And ignore the advertisements that tell you a chocolate bar is a quick energy pick-up. A 30-gram bar of plain milk chocolate has 10 grams of fat, half of them saturated. Pick up an apple instead.

Snack and Fast Foods

Information on the amount and type of fat in the food sold by fast-food and snack chains is not easy to come by. One hamburger chain has a good allergy chart and a booklet listing the ingredients it uses, both available upon request at all its locations. But neither tells you how much fat is in each item. Another hamburger chain has an impressive breakdown of nutritional information for everything it sells, but only if you request it in writing from head office.

A chicken chain can supply only the calories and amount of protein, carbohydrates and total fat in its products. It points out, however, that all this information is subject to change. A submarine sandwich firm can't give a detailed analysis because so much of what it sells comes from other companies.

Consumers' requests for nutritional information are meeting with a bit more success than they once did, mainly because of pressure from Canadians with allergies. But a simple list of ingredients is far from the analysis of total, saturated and unsaturated fat, not to mention sugar content, all of us are entitled to. At the moment, no law requires that this information be posted wherever fast foods are sold.

Until one arrives, you'll just have to use your common sense, and the snack-food section of Appendix 2. You can assume that most fast-food items are high in fat, much of it saturated. You can assume that such things as salad dressings, tartar and mayonnaise-type sauces, and fried or breaded items are best left out of your daily, even weekly, diet and approached as very occasional treats. When you do order them, be sure to ask about the fat content. If enough of us make nuisances of ourselves, we may get some action on disclosure.

Summary

1. Your fat intake should be divided among the saturated, polyunsaturated and mono-unsaturated fats, along the guidelines recommended.
2. There are no "bad" foods, only foods that you shouldn't eat in large quantities.
3. Once you've learned the techniques of cutting fat wherever possible, a low-fat diet will become another good habit.
4. Watch your intake of snack and fast foods in particular; they tend to be very high in fat.

8

Protein

When most people think of protein, they imagine such main course foods as beef, pork, veal, lamb, poultry and fish. And they're quite correct; these taste treats are good sources of protein. But there are many other sources, too.

Remember that cereal commercial? "A serving of cereal X plus four ounces of milk is a good source of dietary protein." Actually, a serving of anything plus four ounces of milk is a good source of dietary protein because the milk is supplying most of it. Although the cereal contributes some protein, by itself it is an incomplete source - as we'll see shortly.

Like carbohydrates and fats, proteins are made from hydrogen, oxygen and carbon atoms. They also contain nitrogen atoms and, depending on the protein, other elements such as sulphur and phosphorous. The building blocks of protein, however, are chemical compounds called amino acids. While there are 22 commonly occurring amino acids - including nine essential ones - hundreds of amino acids can bind together to form a single protein. And some single cells are capable of producing 10,000 different types of protein.

The order of amino acids in the protein is extremely important. A single substitution can be life-threatening. For example, there are 574 amino acids in a single molecule of hemoglobin, an iron-containing protein found in red blood cells. Its primary function is to carry oxygen to the cells of the body. People with sickle cell disease have exactly the same hemoglobin as normal people, with one minor exception: there has been a single substitution of amino acid. That one change results in red blood cells that can appear crescent or sickle-shaped. And owing to that single substitution, those with sickle cell disease may suffer from recurrent attacks of fever, pain in the extremities and other serious symptoms.

Of Prime Importance

Obviously, proteins are necessary for our existence. In fact, the word comes from the Greek *proteios*, meaning of prime importance. Enzymes are proteins, and without enzymes many of the chemical reactions that take place in our bodies would occur so slowly we'd literally die waiting.

We also need protein for the body's growth and repair. Many hormones are proteins, insulin being just one of them. Antibodies are proteins that protect us from infectious disease. Protein is invaluable in maintaining our balance of salt and water, and it helps maintain the pH or acid base balance in the body. Protein can act as a carrier as well. As you learned in an earlier chapter, lipids are transported through the blood wrapped in protein, the complex being called a lipoprotein.

In addition to all the other vital functions protein performs in our bodies, it can be burned to produce energy when necessary. Through chemical reactions, it is metabolized to provide four calories of energy per gram. Those of us who don't eat too much protein won't waste any by turning it into energy. After all, it is too valuable a substance for the body to simply burn. That's a job for fat and the carbohydrates.

The body, in other words, consumes protein as energy only when:

1. We eat more of it than we require.
2. We aren't eating enough carbohydrate and/or fat.
3. We can't build the proteins we need with the amino acids that are in our cells.

How Much Protein Do We Need?

The amount of protein each of us requires is based on age, sex and desirable body weight (not actual). The average healthy adult should be getting only enough amino acids to replace existing body stores of protein. Children and pregnant women need enough to allow for both replacement and the manufacture of additional body protein for growth purposes.

Rather than getting involved in calculating grams of protein per kilogram of weight, or performing nitrogen balance studies on human beings, experts have concluded that you'll be quite safe if only 15 to 20 per cent of the calories you require come from protein. However, the Canadian Consensus Conference has recommended that those with elevated blood lipids limit their protein intake to 10 to 15 per cent of daily calories. Part of the reason, of course, is that protein can be high in dietary fat, a point we'll get to shortly.

You'll note that these percentages are based on the calories you require to maintain a desirable weight for your sex, age and height. We're not talking 10 or 20 per cent of the calories you actually eat in a day, which may be far more than you need.

Complete and Incomplete Protein

Not all foods contain complete proteins; they lack some essential amino acid or are low in others. Generally speaking, protein derived from animals is complete. That means that dairy products, eggs, meat, fish and poultry are excellent sources of all the essential and non-essential amino acids.

Protein from the vegetable and fruit world tends to be incomplete, and that's one reason why it's so important to eat a variety of foods. Strict vegetarians have to very carefully combine protein sources to ensure that each meal furnishes them with enough of the essential amino acids. For example, the essential ones in which grains are low are abundant in legumes. Thus by combining cornbread and pinto beans, you can correct the amino acid deficiency that would exist if you ate only corn (a grain) or beans.

In general, to get complete protein you must eat legumes (including peanuts) with either grains, nuts or seeds; rice with either wheat, legumes, seeds or nuts; and wheat with either legumes, nuts, seeds or rice. Remember that nuts, seeds and peanuts contain a lot of fat, even though it is unsaturated.

Table 8.1 Complementary Proteins

To get complete protein, you must eat combinations like these at the same meal.

Legumes	plus	*Grains*
Dried beans	+	Barley
Peas	+	Millet
Lentils	+	Rice
Soybeans	+	Oats
Soybean curd (tofu)	+	Brown rice
Mung beans	+	Rye
Split peas	+	Cornmeal
Garbanzo beans	+	Bulgar (cracked wheat)
Peanuts	+	Wheat

Legumes	plus	*Nuts and Seeds*
as above	+	Almonds, brazil nuts
		cashews, pecans, walnuts,
		pumpkin seeds, sesame
		seeds, sunflower seeds

Grains	plus	*Nuts, Seeds or Legumes*
Rice	+	Sesame seeds or cashews
Wheat germ	+	Peanuts
Corn	+	Soybeans
Noodles	+	Cashews
Wheat bread	+	Peanut butter

Vegetables	plus	*Legumes, Grains*
Dark green leafy	+	Pinto beans
Stir-fried vegetables	+	Kidney beans
Broccoli	+	Corn over brown rice
Potatoes	+	Corn

The Problem of Too Much Protein

As valuable as protein is, exceeding your requirements may be harmful. For starters, you're not eating only protein. High-protein foods like red meat often contain significant amounts of fat, much of it hidden from sight. Thus, eating lots of protein-rich food will increase your fat intake. It's also certain to increase the number of calories you consume, and that won't help you reach or maintain your ideal weight.

There are other reasons to avoid over-consumption. The body uses enzymes, vitamins and minerals to process proteins. Too much protein may cause deficiencies or shortages of these substances. Too much may also cause an increase in zinc excretion and deplete our bodies of calcium. Too much can even cause dehydration. Our bodies must break down any excess protein for storage. This involves removing its nitrogen, which then has to be excreted. Because that involves diluting it in the urine, our water requirements increase.

Athletic types in particular must watch out for this problem. They tend to overeat protein and, given their sweating and other types of water loss, they already may be verging on dehydration. The extra water loss from protein excretion may push them over the edge, especially in warm weather.

Protein Facts and Fancies

Some people buy protein supplements; others buy amino acid supplements. Neither purchase is necessary. Supplements are required only by those who for some reason are unable to eat a balanced diet. If you can eat, you can get all the protein you need from food. Not only that, a balanced diet will give you complete protein and essential amino acids, as well as all the vitamins, minerals and trace nutrients your body requires to process and utilize the proteins.

A high-protein diet won't make your muscles bulge, either. For that, you need a balanced diet, vigorous exercise and training. Nor will taking protein supplements improve your skin, nails or hair, unless you're protein-deficient. In this country that's virtually impossible. The average Canadian gets too much rather than too little protein.

For example, a cup of milk, half a cup of vegetables, three ounces of meat and a slice of bread add up to 34 grams of protein. That's more than half the 61 grams a middle-aged man needs in a day. It's almost the total 44-gram requirement of a middle-aged woman. And that was only lunch. An egg, cup of milk and slice

Table 8.2 How Protein Affects Blood Cholesterol

Lowers	No Effect	Increases
Fatty fish (salmon, sardine, mackerel, kippers, herring, pilchard, trout) Non-fat milk Buttermilk	Other fish Lean meat and meat by-products in reasonable amounts Lean poultry (chicken, turkey) without skin Eggs (in some people) Seafood (shrimp, scallops, clams)	Meat and meat by-products in excessive amounts especially if fat-marbled or untrimmed Fatty fowl (goose and duck) Eggs (in some people) Poultry with skin Cream Whole and 2% milk Butter

of dry toast for breakfast would add another 17 grams. Need we go on?

The additional problem, of course, is all the fat a diet like this represents, particularly if the milk is whole rather than skim. Animal proteins are likely to contain mainly saturated fat, while plant proteins usually have predominately mono- or polyunsaturated lipids. As well, plant sources have far less fat in general.

So when it comes to main courses, the prudent eater makes such things as vegetables and legumes the stars, with meat and other animal proteins playing a very minor supporting role. After all, Chinese-style cuisine can feed four people well on less than half a pound of meat.

Summary

1. Proteins are essential nutrients.
2. We require a balanced diet to manufacture our own proteins.
3. Most Canadians eat too much protein, and that can be harmful because of the usually high fat content.
4. Animal proteins tend to contain significant amounts of saturated fats, whereas vegetable protein sources are less likely to contain hidden fat.

5. Vegetable sources may be more desirable because they usually contain mono- and polyunsaturated fats, but they do not supply complete protein.
6. To make plant sources complete, one protein source must be complemented by another to ensure all essential amino acids are included in the same meal (see Table 8.1).

9

Carbohydrates

When most of us think about carbohydrates we see cake, candy, honey, sugar and other sweet things. All that bad stuff. But, oh, so good-tasting, at least to those of us with sweet tooths. We can almost feel our waistlines getting bigger with every bite.

Actually, we'd be more on target scientifically if we associated carbohydrates with the sun. Without that big ball of burning gas that lights and heats the world, there would be no carbohydrates. That's because the best food sources come from plants. In a process called photosynthesis, the earth's foliage uses carbon dioxide gas from the air, water from the soil and energy from the sun to make carbohydrates. The word itself means hydrated or watered carbons.

What's important to us as eaters, however, is that every wonderful gram has only four calories, versus nine for fats. Yet it's carbohydrates that have a reputation for being "fattening."

Contrary to popular belief, the "starchy" foods - potatoes, corn, bread, pasta and such - are anything but fattening. They're what used to be called "rib-sticking" foods. They make us feel fuller for a longer period of time. And because of that satisfaction, we tend to eat less, keeping us thinner.

The Canadian Consensus Conference panel recommended that those with elevated lipids get the majority of their daily calories from carbohydrates: 55 to 60 per cent. There should also be, it said, an emphasis on a variety of foods containing dietary fibre. We'll get to fibre and the complex carbohydrates shortly. First, let's deal with the simple ones - the sugars.

The Simple Carbohydrates

There are sugars and there are sugars, with many different names. Glucose, fructose, mannose and galactose, for example. In chemistry, two such simple sugars joined can make a third. Join a glucose with a fructose and you get sucrose. Two glucoses joined make maltose. A glucose and galactose yield a lactose.

You've probably heard of some of these sugars, or read their names on food labels. Glucose, also known as dextrose, grape sugar and corn sugar, occurs naturally in fruits and such vegetables as fresh corn and carrots. It's the sugar that doctors normally measure in your blood and check for in your urine. The cells of our bodies use glucose as a source of energy; in fact, it's our major source, fuelling both brain and muscles.

Fructose, or fruit sugar, is found naturally in fruit and honey and is the sweetest of the common sugars. Mannitol is derived from mannose and eating too much of it may give you diarrhea.

Sorbitol is a derivative of glucose with about the same sweetness but the advantage that our guts absorb it into the bloodstream less quickly. In essence, then, it can give you a slower charge than glucose while tasting just as good and ultimately supplying the same number of calories. Another sugar, xylitol, occurs naturally in fruits and some vegetables.

Xylitol, sorbitol and mannitol are actually classified as sugar alcohols. While products containing them are sometimes labelled "sugar free," gram for gram they have just as many calories as sugar. Xylitol has been used as an alternative sweetener in such products as chewing gum because bacteria in the mouth don't thrive on it and, theoretically, it should cause fewer cavities than sugar. Indeed, some studies have suggested that it may actually suppress the growth of bacteria that produce dental cavities. Just remember that if swallowed it may not save you any calories.

Lactose or milk sugar is a carbohydrate that doesn't come from a plant. Cow's milk is 4.5 per cent lactose; human milk contains 75 per cent. To utilize lactose our bodies have to break it down into glucose and galactose, a process that requires an enzyme called lactase. Some people have a deficiency of this enzyme and hence can't tolerate milk products.

The Refined and Processed Sugars

Table sugar, the white granulated stuff most of us shovel into coffee and toss on cereal, is sucrose refined from sugar cane and sugar beets. Sucrose is also found in some fruits and vegetables. Brown sugar is white sugar coloured by the addition of molasses. Molasses is a syrup left over when sucrose is refined from cane sugar. Corn syrup is produced when enzymes break cornstarch into a mixture that's mostly glucose with some maltose. Maple sugar is mostly sucrose and comes from the sap of the maple tree. Real maple syrup is a luxury few of us can afford; the substitutes we pour over pancakes and waffles are likely sucrose solutions with artificial maple flavour added.

The crystals of raw sugar, that grainy brown mixture you see in fancy restaurants, are formed from concentrated sugar cane juice. They're tan or brown simply because the manufacturing process that makes sugar white hasn't been completed. Even so, raw sugar is more expensive than plain white table sugar.

There are a few other names you may notice on food labels or packages. Invert sugar is a mixture of glucose and fructose in liquid form. Sweeter than sucrose, it can be used to prevent crystallization in candy and ice cream. Malt sugar is maltose, which doesn't form naturally; fermenting grain adds it to beer and it's also found in some processed cereals and baby foods.

When it comes to sweetness, sucrose (granulated sugar) is the standard to which the others are compared. Fructose is about 70 per cent sweeter; invert sugar about 30 per cent sweeter. On the other side of the scale, glucose is about 25 per cent less sweet than sucrose, while lactose, the least sweet of the common sugars, has about 15 per cent of sucrose's sweetness.

Rating the Simple Sugars

Which sugar is better? That depends on what you mean by better. For one thing, they're all carbohydrates so, from a calorie point of view, they all supply about four calories per gram. For another, granulated sugar is a lot cheaper than maple syrup. Some people seem to feel fructose is more natural than glucose, or pass up sucrose for the much more expensive fructose on the grounds that they'll use less of it because it's sweeter. However, we burn calories by metabolizing the foods we eat. And to metabolize glucose we burn *more* calories than we do for a similar quantity of fructose. So in the end, fructose actually may be more fattening.

Others insist that honey, a combination of glucose and fructose, is better for us than granulated sugar. Both are natural carbohydrates; it's simply that honey is more expensive. And because a teaspoon of gooey honey weighs considerably more than one of granulated sugar, you're getting extra calories. In fact, almost double the number: 22 vs 13. There goes another notch on your belt. Not only that, at least one group of researchers found that some honey samples contained possible cancer-promoting substances.

If you want truly natural sugar, eat vegetables and fruits and drink milk. When you do, you're getting some nutrients instead of empty calories. Why not spend your money on something useful? To see just how empty some calories can be, let's take a look at the nutrients in a few common foods, as shown in Tables 9.1 and 9.2. As you'll notice, pure sugars like sucrose or honey, and such sugary products as cola-type drinks, supply you with concentrated energy but virtually no other nutrients. Orange juice, skim milk and vegetables, however, are full of the elements you need to stay healthy.

If you don't already, take the time to check the ingredient listings on any packaged products you buy. Ingredients are listed in order of quantity, with the most heavily used first on the list. If you see sugar or anything ending in "ose" near or at the top of the list, you'd be wise to seek out another product.

The Complex Carbohydrates

Complex carbohydrates are made up of many, many simple sugars. The starch found in cereal grains, vegetables, tubers and legumes, for example, is made up of about 3,000 glucose molecules. When we eat this starch, enzymes in the saliva and gut break it down into glucose so that it can be absorbed into the bloodstream.

But while our bodies ultimately return the starch to its original form as glucose, there is a time lag. The process of absorption into the blood is delayed, and this is what makes these complex sugars particularly useful. When we eat simple sugars, absorption can occur right away, with no processing by the enzymes in our mouths and guts. This causes a sudden elevation in blood sugar, which can lead to a surge in the secretion of insulin. And this, in turn, can make us hungry more quickly, something of which the complex carbohydrates can't be accused.

Some parts of complex carbohydrates can't be processed at all by our digestive systems. The yellow skin on corn niblets, those strings of celery that get caught in your teeth, and the inner skin-like membranes that separate an orange into segments, all come out of our bodies in the same form they went in.

Yet these portions are also valuable members of the wonderful world of dietary fibre. You may know it as roughage, or have seen references to crude fibre. It's all fibre, and most of us don't eat enough of it. We'll get to that point later; right now, let's look at some of the various types of dietary fibre, starting with two that are not soluble in water.

The Dietary Fibres

Cellulose is the most plentiful complex sugar found in plants. Because it attracts water in our colons, eating it gives us bulkier, more watery stools. It may give us some gas, too: our gut enzymes can't digest it, but the bacteria in our colons can cause it to ferment. Cellulose is found in broccoli, cabbage, carrots, lima beans, peanuts, pears, peas, wax beans and whole wheat flour.

Hemicellulose, which is made up of glucose, xylose and mannose, also attracts water to the stool and can be digested by gut bacteria. It's present in bananas, beets, eggplant, radishes and sweet corn. Both cellulose and hemicellulose are found in apples, bran and whole wheat cereals, brussels sprouts and green beans.

Two fibres that are water-soluble are thought to be of special help in cholesterol control. Pectin, a fibre food that anyone who's made jam will recognize, forms a gel when mixed with water. It's found naturally in fruits and vegetables. The gums and mucilages dissolve in water. Guar gum, locust bean gum, carob gum and gum arabic are used to thicken and mix commercial food products, but are found naturally in oatmeal, oat bran and legumes.

Table 9.1 Comparative Nutritional Analysis of Some Carbohydrate Foods

	Granulated Sugar	Strained Liquid Honey	Regular Cola Drink
Measure	1 tbsp.	1 tbsp.	280 mL
	(15 mL)	(15 mL)	
Calories	50	64	120
Protein (g)	0	trace	0
Carbohydrates (g)	13	17	30
Fat (g)	0	0	0
SFA (g)	0	0	0
PUFA (g)	0	0	0
Cholesterol (mg)	0	0	0
Calcium (mg)	0	1	9
Iron (mg)	.2	.1	trace
Sodium (mg)	2	1	12
Potassium (mg)	6	11	3
Vitamin A (RE)	0	0	0
Thiamin (mg)	0	trace	0
Riboflavin (mg)	0	trace	0
Niacin (NE)	0	trace	0
Foliate (mcg)	-	trace	0
Vitamin C (mg)	0	trace	0
Dietary fibre (g)	-	-	-

From *Nutrient Value of Some Common Foods*, Health and Welfare Canada, 1988

Lignin is the woody material in stems and bark. While some sources suggest that eating it helps keep blood cholesterols low, most folks wouldn't find it very appetizing. By rights, it really isn't a fibre.

Why Carbohydrates are So Important

As we've seen, there are hazards associated with the overconsumption of both fats and proteins. That leaves carbohydrates as the ideal source of calories. Complex carbohydrates are satiating,

**Table 9.2 Comparative Nutritional Analysis
of Some Carbohydrate Foods**

	Fresh Orange Juice	Skim Milk	Apple[1]	Potato[2]
Measure	1 cup (250mL)	1 cup (250mL)	medium	2-3/4 in. (7cm) long
Calories	118	90	81	116
Protein (g)	2	9	trace	2
Carbohydrates (g)	27	13	21	27
Fat (g)	trace	trace	trace	trace
SFA (g)	trace	trace	trace	trace
PUFA (g)	trace	trace	trace	trace
Cholesterol (mg)	0	5	0	0
Calcium (mg)	29	320	10	11
Iron (mg)	5	.1	.2	.4
Sodium (mg)	3	133	0	7
Potassium (mg)	524	429	159	443
Vitamin A (RE)	52	158	7	0
Thiamin (mg)	.24	.09	.02	.13
Riboflavin (mg)	.08	.36	.02	.03
Niacin (NE)	1.1	2.3	.2	2.4
Foliate (mcg)	79	13	4	12
Vitamin C (mg)	131	3	8	10
Dietary fibre (g)	1.0	-	3.5	1.4

[1] Raw with skin.
[2] Peeled before boiling.

From *Nutrient Value of Some Common Foods*, Health and Welfare Canada, 1988

relatively inexpensive, and they don't raise cholesterol levels. We should all be consuming potatoes, pasta, rice and other starch-rich foods.

While the news that complex carbohydrates aren't fattening may come as a surprise, we've all heard about the health benefits of fibre. Because it's not digested and absorbed, fibre makes the stool bulky. And that keeps the bowels moving, preventing constipation. Studies have shown that high-volume stools and a speedy intestinal transit time (the time it takes for food to go from mouth through gut to toilet) lead to good bowel health.

A high-fibre diet is thought to decrease the risk of gallstones, appendicitis, diverticulosis, hemorrhoids, varicose veins and cancer of the colon, as a result of its ability to keep the bowels moving and the effect that has on colonic bacteria. Non-water-soluble (insoluble) fibre binds with fats and sterols present in the gut. As a result these substances, including cholesterol, are excreted with the stool instead of being absorbed by the gut. At least that's the theory. In practice, wheat bran, which contains a lot of insoluble fibre, has not been shown to lower blood cholesterol. On the other hand, oat bran, which is a good source of soluble fibre, does lower blood cholesterol. The "how" isn't known. Perhaps there's something present that interferes with cholesterol production or increases its excretion. No one knows for certain.

More predictably than its effects on cholesterol, dietary fibre exerts a positive effect on how our guts handle glucose. The fibre seems to help us regulate our blood glucose levels and the effect is long-lasting. (A high-fibre breakfast can still exert its effects at lunchtime.) It's so effective that diabetics may be able to reduce their pill dosage or insulin when they switch to a high-fibre diet.

As with all foods, variety is important with fibre. Fruits, vegetables, legumes, wheat bran, nuts, seeds, popcorn, whole grain flours and rice are all sources of insoluble cellulose and hemicellulose fibre. They are important in keeping your transit time fast and preventing constipation. However, in too great a quantity they might interfere with the absorption of minerals.

The water-soluble fibres like pectins and gums are found in fruits, vegetables, seeds, legumes, oats, barley and rye. They are more effective in lowering blood cholesterol but not as effective in increasing transit time or preventing constipation.

None of the official dietary guidelines tell us how much fibre to consume, but that may well change. Part of the problem is that there is some disagreement as to how fibre should be measured. Most experts suggest 20 to 30 grams of dietary fibre per day, but they do not differentiate between soluble and insoluble types. (See Appendix 3 for listings of fibre content.)

Specific Fruits and Vegetables

A number of fruits and vegetables have been reported to have a beneficial effect on cholesterol levels. Many of the reports are anecdotal; others are not based on the best scientific methods. Perhaps someday we'll be more certain. In the meantime, here's what information is available.

Apples: Two to three apples a day may lower cholesterol and slightly raise HDLs, reduce blood pressure and keep blood sugar levels steady.

Banana and plantain: Like apples, bananas contain pectin and may lower blood cholesterol. Unripe plantain (it looks like a large green banana even when ripe) seemed to counteract the effects of increased dietary cholesterol and raised HDL levels when fed to rats.

Barley: Eating barley or foods made with it has been shown in human studies to lower blood cholesterol by about 15 per cent.

Beans: A cup or less of cooked pinto or navy beans a day was shown in one study to appreciably lower LDLs.

Carrots: One study reported that 2-1/2 medium-size carrots a day lowered cholesterol by 11 per cent.

Currants: In animal experiments, chemicals in currants (anthocyanosides) have some beneficial effects on blood vessels.

Eggplant: Some studies have suggested that eggplant may inhibit the rise in blood cholesterol caused by other foods.

Garlic and onion: Buy lots of these. Cooking with them can liven up a bland menu, and both seem to show anti-coagulant activity in a number of studies.

Ginger: This spice may have some effect on lowering blood cholesterol.

Grapefruit: The pectin in the pulp (not in the juice) has been studied for its cholesterol-lowering value. Volunteers fed 15 grams of grapefruit pectin a day for four months had an average drop of 8 per cent in their cholesterol levels, and some had increased HDLs. How many grapefruit add up to 15 grams of pectin has not yet been figured out: something between two and 15, perhaps. Orange pectin may share the same properties.

Mushrooms: Not the little white ones you buy at supermarkets but shiittake, a brown oriental mushroom, and Chinese tree ear may help lower blood cholesterol. (Actually, mushrooms are not vegetables. They're not even plants; they're fungi.)

The Wonders of Oat Bran

Until recently, only mothers seemed to like hot oat cereal. All that changed when it was discovered that oat bran contained some ingredient that lowered blood cholesterol. No one is sure exactly how it works, but there seems to be pretty good agreement that it does.

In one study where 140 grams of rolled oats were incorporated into the daily bread, cholesterol levels fell 11 per cent after three weeks. (Rolled oats are about half oat bran.) In two other studies cholesterols were lowered 13 and 19 per cent respectively by eating 100 grams of oat bran per day.

A couple of researchers came up with a dose-response formula for oat bran's cholesterol-lowering effects. If you multiply the amount of oat bran consumed in grams by 0.156, then add one, that is the percentage your cholesterol will be lowered on average. So 100 grams per day should lower your cholesterol 16.6 per cent.

There is a danger here. By establishing a dose-response equation, oat bran has been turned into a drug. Don't fool yourself into believing that because it is a "natural" drug, it's safe. Digitalis, belladona and arsenic are natural drugs; all of them can kill at inappropriate doses.

People have a tendency to figure that if 35 grams of something is good, 100 grams is better and 350 is better still. Naturally, we're smart enough to realize this is not true. Too much of a good thing may be quite detrimental. Don't get sucked into the oat bran craze. It's likely that we know much more about the side effects of such cholesterol-lowering drugs as cholestyramine than we do about oat bran.

A typical serving of oat bran is one ounce or about 35 grams dry weight. A 100-gram dry weight is a pretty hefty serving. It's not reasonable to exceed 50 to 100 grams per day unless you do so under some form of medical supervision. And since rolled oats are cheaper and easier to find on the supermarket shelf, they may be a preferable source of oat bran.

Alcohol and Caffeine

There was some evidence to suggest that alcohol in moderation might actually protect against coronary heart disease and raise HDL cholesterol. However, more recent research has cast some doubt on this theory. Alcohol also raises triglycerides. Most experts suggest that alcohol in moderation - one or two drinks a day - is not harmful. Everyone agrees that any more than that is harmful.

Depending on your preference, alcoholic drinks may be high in sugar and calories. Best choices are dry wines, dry sherries and light beers. More fattening are wines with a sugar rating of 3 or over, regular beer and liqueurs.

Choose mixes that are low in sugar or sugar-free, such as water, diet soft drinks, mineral water, soda or tomato juice.

Caffeine is found in coffee, tea, chocolate and cola drinks (and even in such medications as cold remedies, headache relievers and weight control aids). Evidence linking caffeine to coronary artery disease is conflicting, but moderation is wise. Three to four cups of average-strength coffee or strongly brewed tea contain about 450 mg of caffeine. A cola drink has half the caffeine of a cup of coffee.

A prudent person might consider that one or two cups of coffee or caffeine equivalent during the day, plus an alcoholic drink at dinner, is a reasonable amount. That's not to say that either are recommended.

Table 9.3 How Carbohydrates Affect Blood Cholesterol

Lowers	No Effect	Increases
Oat bran	Wheat bran	Sucrose (table sugar)
Fruits and	Soybean fibre	Fructose (fruit sugar)
vegetables with	Starch	
soluble fibre	Glucose	
(pectin, gums)	Cellulose fibre	
or hemicellulose		
Legumes		
Alfalfa		
Barley, oats and		
other grains		
Soy milk		

What You Now Know About Food

Now that you're reaching the end of four chapters on food, let's sum up what you know. For a start, you know you have to pay attention to cutting back on protein, fat, simple sugars and calories. If you consume more than two alcoholic drinks or caffeine equivalents a day, that needs reducing as well.

What can you eat lots of? Complex carbohydrates like pasta, potatoes and rice, plus high fibre foods like oat and wheat bran, fruits and vegetables.

You know you can avoid empty sugar calories and excess fat by limiting your consumption of processed and packaged foods, especially those that have butter, margarine, shortening, vegetable oils, sugar and anything that ends with "ose" (like sucrose) high on their lists of ingredients. You'll go out of your way to avoid highly saturated fats, including palm, palm kernel and coconut oils, as well as unnatural hydrogenated vegetable oils.

You won't be impressed by advertising claims that some non-animal food product is "cholesterol free" because you know that vegetable sources don't contain cholesterol. Unless your doctor tells you otherwise, you're not even going to concentrate on the cholesterol content of what you eat because it's the SFAs, the saturated fatty acids, that are more important in raising cholesterol.

You know that all fats are especially rich in calories, a big nine calories a gram. And while you're going to limit your fat content as much as you can within reason, you'll be sure to get a combination of foods that provide you with roughly equal amounts of SFA, MUFA and PUFA in a day.

You understand that while protein intake may have to be cut, you require a full complement of amino acid building blocks each day. You also realize that foods high in protein tend to be high-cost foods, so saving money is another good reason to cut back on them. Finally, you know that high-protein foods like meat have hidden fat in them. And that increases both your calories and your saturated fat intake.

Summary

1. Carbohydrates are the ideal energy food.
2. Choose complex carbohydrates in natural form, like fruits and vegetables, over refined sugars.
3. Since the ideal amount of dietary fibre has yet to be determined, don't go overboard.
4. Eat a variety of high-fibre foods to ensure that you get both soluble and insoluble fibre.

10

Weight, Exercise, Personality & Stress

This chapter covers the other components of your lifestyle that may affect your blood cholesterol in particular or your chances of developing heart and other diseases generally. We'll start with determining your ideal weight.

Expert advice on lifestyle and prevention always seems to include a recommendation to either reduce down to or eat up to and then maintain your "ideal" weight. What the professionals fail to provide, however, is a definition of ideal weight.

On the surface, their lack of guidelines shouldn't provide much of a problem. All you need to do is hunt around for a table of ideal weights and compare yourself. We received permission to reprint one such popular table but opted not to reproduce it. You see, comparing yourself to a chart may not be all that worthwhile.

For starters, aside from compensating for your state of dress and the height of the heels on your shoes, you really should calculate your frame size by measuring things like elbow breadth. It's all very cumbersome. Anyway, how important is it to compare yourself to a bunch of people who have bought life insurance from a specified group of insurance companies? Particularly when some of the heights and weights put on applications for life insurance are "estimated."

Now that we've discounted the tables for being unscientific, we can't very well tell you to use the old-fashioned rule of thumb: for men, start with 110 pounds for the first five feet of height and add five pounds for every inch over that (5-foot-10, then, would translate to 10 x 5 + 110 = 160 pounds). For women, start with 100 pounds and do the same (5-foot-4 translates to 4 x 5 + 100 = 120 pounds). No, even though these guesstimates involve complicated two-step mathematics, the results just aren't sophisticated enough for the late 20th century.

Those of you who belong to a fancy, expensive health club are frothing at the mouth with the answer. Your fitness and lifestyle consultant has explained to you that height and weight are such "crude" measurements. After all, they don't measure fatness.Everyone knows that lean muscle is denser than fat, which means it weighs more. So a very muscular football player may be overweight, even obese, when judged by a height-weight measurement. But he is unlikely to be fat. Scales and measuring tapes may be fine for the disadvantaged. For you as a special member, however, measuring fatness is much more appropriate.

Measuring Lean Body Mass

There are, of course, very scientific ways of measuring lean body mass. A simple but accurate one is to measure the amount of water that you displace when you're submersed in a tank. Your density (weight per volume) can then be calculated and your leanness or fatness estimated. Trouble is, the procedure can be messy and most of us don't have specially designed water tanks available. Anyway, we know what happened to Houdini when he played around with tankfuls of water.

No matter, the pros at your club can estimate fatness by measuring fatfold thickness with calipers, those compass-like instruments that look like the things navigators use. With these instruments measurements are taken on the back of the upper arm, below the shoulder blade or in other imaginative places, then compared to tables divided into columns based on age and sex. This is obviously a better way to determine ideal weight. The calipers are expensive, only rarely are such measurements done by doctors, and the entire process is much more sophisticated than stripping down and standing on a scale.

The thing is, though, an accurate weigh scale yields accurate and reproducible weights. All you need do is stand on it. Even accurately calibrated fatfold calipers may produce less accurate or reproducible measurements, particularly if they're performed by an inexperienced or untrained person. But that's not all. Fat isn't evenly dispersed over the body: the amount a person has may be different in different areas. Some people tend to get fatter in their bellies than anywhere else. And a number of reports have suggested that those with fat bellies are at greater risk of heart disease and other health problems than those who have most of their fat elsewhere. The Canadian Consensus panel, in fact, said that "obesity, particularly abdominal obesity" puts patients in the priority group for blood lipid testing.

Having dismissed all the common methods for determining ideal weight as being less than ideal, what's left? You could peel down and take a gander in a full-length mirror. If what you see looks too fat, then it's likely that you're above your ideal weight. Trouble is, many people have distorted ideas of what their weights should be and how they should look. So if you opt for the mirror test, perhaps you should first obtain a certificate from a psychiatrist saying you don't suffer from an eating disorder.

Calculating Your Body Mass Index

Don't despair. There is another way. And although it does have limitations, it doesn't require calipers, tanks of water or a psychiatric consultation. It's called the Body Mass Index, or BMI for short. Here's how to do it.

- Take your weight in kilograms (if your scale only weighs in pounds, divide by 2.2 to get kilograms)   _____(A)
- Take your height in metres (if you have it in inches, multiply by 0.025 to convert to metres)   _____(B)
- Square your height in metres by multiplying (B) by (B)   _____(C)
- Divide (A) by (C) to get your Body Mass Index or BMI

Let's calculate the BMI for a person who's 155 pounds and 5-foot-6.

- Divide the weight in pounds (155) by 2.2   = 70.5 kg
- Height in inches (66) times 0.025   = 1.65 metres
- Square the height by multiplying
  1.65 x 1.65   = 2.7 metres
- Divide the weight in kg by the
  height in metres squared
  (70.5 divided by 2.7)   = 26.1 kg/m²

Thank goodness for pocket calculators! But what's a normal BMI? Ideal is 22.4 for women and 22.7 for men. If you define overweight as being 20 per cent greater than ideal, the numbers are 26.9 for women and 27.2 for men. You are 40 per cent over ideal if your BMI is 31.4 for women and 31.8 for men. A BMI of 20 or less may signify that you're underweight, which in some circumstances can be associated with health problems.

As imperfect and open to criticism as it may be, the BMI seems to be the preferred method of gauging ideal weight this year. Take a couple of minutes to calculate yours.

Controlling Your Weight

The weight of your body follows a simple equation: energy (calories) in minus energy (activity) out = change in body fat reserves. Actually, we expend calories when we're inactive, too, but that complicates the equation.

A pound of fat represents 3,500 calories. Eat 3,500 more than you spend and you'll gain a pound. Eat 3,500 fewer than you require for your activity level and you'll lose a pound. At 500 fewer calories a day, that pound would be gone in a week.

A slow and steady weight loss is far better for you than the abrupt changes of any fad diet. Most experts recommend that you lose no more than two or three pounds a week. Cutting your calories by 1,000 a day would take off two pounds in a week and additional exercise could account for a bit more.

How do you figure out how many calories you need for an ordinary, non-dieting day? Well, you could turn to Table 7.1 in the chapter on dietary fats. But what is average? Some calorie requirements are calculated on the assumption that you sit for seven hours a day, stand for five, walk for two, do light physical activity for another two, and sleep for eight. Obviously, not everyone falls into that specific a lifestyle.

There are some extremely complicated ways to find out the exact number of calories you require given your rate of metabolism and your activity level. The simplest way, however, is to just pay attention to what works for you. If you're putting on weight or are unable to lose any, it's clear that you're eating too much and/or not getting enough exercise.

Why We Overeat

Why some people overeat and others undereat is a complicated and often ill-understood area. As with many other components of nature, the answers are not simple. We all know people who seem to put away enormous amounts of food and yet can't gain weight. And then there are others who claim that all they need to do is look at food and they gain weight. To consider all the theories and facts would require another book. Here are a few generalizations.

For starters, most weight problems are *not* related to hormonal imbalances. The majority of overweight people are not deficient in thyroid hormone, growth hormone or any other hormone. Nor are the majority of underweight people suffering from overactive endocrine glands. This does not mean that people with weight problems and symptoms suggestive of other imbalances should not be tested for hormonal disorders. In the vast majority of instances, however, the tests will be normal.

Many if not the vast majority of eating problems, whether they be eating too much or too little, are the result of behavioural disorders. Viewed in this way, the eating problem is then a symptom of something else, such as anxiety or depression. As a result, treating your weight by going on a diet to gain or reduce is like taking a headache tablet because one of your fingers is caught in vise grip pliers. Although the painkiller is in your system and the pain might be lessened, your finger is still being squeezed in the vise. The same holds true for dieting. You may gain or lose the weight necessary to get you to your ideal, but because the anxiety, depression or other behavioural problem persists, the weight problem returns in time.

There is little doubt that differences between people partially account for our final weights. Some of these differences may be inherited. Others are learned. Some are physiological. There may be others over which we have no voluntary control. What is apparent, and it has been proven over and over again, is that fad diets have no lasting benefit for the vast majority of those who attempt them. Many are expensive and simply not worth the money. Others are frankly dangerous to your health. Some involving injections of hormones and vitamins are absolutely useless.

The prudent diet recommended by the Canadian Heart and Stroke Foundation and others guarantees you adequate nutrition. With some expert assistance, perhaps from your doctor, a registered dietitian, nurse or other health care professional, a prudent diet can be tailored to your particular needs. Not only will this sort of diet help you reach and maintain your ideal weight, it will also ensure that your blood cholesterol remains in a healthy range.

We have made light of the entire concept of "ideal" weight because no one has adequately defined it, and because you are an individual with your own personal needs. No one should make you feel guilty because a chart suggests you should weigh 70 kg and you weigh 75 or 80. We have to be reasonable. Unless you are suffering from some psychiatric problem that affects your ability to reasonably assess your ideal weight by looking in a mirror, listening to the comments of your peers and spouse, and judging how you feel in your clothes and during physical activity, you'll know what your ideal weight is *without* having to refer to a table or calculate your BMI. In other words, if you are reasonably well adjusted and you feel too fat, you likely are. Get an impartial opinion from your doctor, then discuss a strategy to deal with your weight problem - if indeed you have one.

Finally, not everyone who is overweight has an elevated cholesterol, high blood pressure, varicose veins, arthritis, diabetes or any of the other conditions that may be associated with obesity. However, if you do suffer from any weight-related disorders, like an elevated blood cholesterol, dieting down to an ideal weight may well cure your problem.

Studies on Exercise

The consensus on regular aerobic exercise is that at the very least, it makes people feel better. Beyond that, for the present time, we'd be on sort of shaky ground to make claims. Part of the problem is that human beings have good intentions for rather short periods of time. We'll join a fitness club and go at an exercise program gung ho for weeks or months, but few of us persist on a regular basis for much longer than that. The same holds true of individuals who enter studies to measure the benefits of physical fitness. Due to high drop-out rates and problems with study design and data collection, it is difficult to draw firm conclusions. No matter, we'll look at trends. But, first, a few study examples may give you an idea of the difficulties.

The double-decker buses that London, England, is famous for are manned by a driver who spends his time sitting and a conductor whose job is more physically active. In comparing the two groups, the conductors had 30 per cent fewer symptoms of heart disease and 50 per cent fewer heart attacks than the sedentary drivers. The conclusion seems obvious: being physically active is good for your heart. However, when it came to angina (chest pain caused by coronary artery disease), the conductors suffered about twice as much. And as a later study showed, there may have been more to it than what the men did during their working hours. When the records of the men at the time of hiring were examined, those who were to become drivers had waists at least an inch greater and higher blood cholesterols and blood pressures than those who ended up being conductors. So, in the end, it is hard to draw any sort of meaningful conclusion.

Similar studies were done with other groups, such as inside versus outside postal workers. Others have looked at weekend activities of white collar workers, of Harvard University alumni and of California longshoremen. Overall, the results suggested that being physically active, even mildly so, was better for the heart than being sedentary. Thus, walking a few extra blocks or climbing stairs instead of taking the elevator appears to give the hearts of men some extra degree of protection. Another interesting suggestion that has surfaced from examining athletes was that the benefits of physical activity were not long-lasting. The protective effect ceased when regular activity did.

There is evidence showing that for both men and women, the better physical shape one is in, the lower the resting heart rate, body weight, blood pressure, blood cholesterol, blood trigly-cerides, blood sugar and per cent body fat. In addition, physical fitness apparently increases the protective HDL cholesterol. Nonetheless, some studies have been published suggesting that not all of these factors are influenced by exercise. And even if the differences are real, perhaps it is not the exercise that is making the difference. After all, people of a certain personality type may be the ones who indulge in endurance-type exercise over prolonged periods of time. Or perhaps those who exercise regularly take better overall care of themselves - they eat less saturated fat, total fat and salt, and don't smoke. Perhaps the exercise is an outlet for tension and anxiety, resulting in less heart disease.

Nowadays there are numerous cardiac rehabilitation programs for those who suffer from angina, have had heart attacks, or who have had by-pass surgery. Some individuals in these programs do very well. Those who stick with the programs likely feel better. And because of the follow-up a participant will be more likely to take care of his or her entire lifestyle, not just the exercise component of it. But unfortunately, although we all have a gut feeling that these programs decrease the symptoms and prolong the lives of at least some of the participants, it is difficult to prove scientifically. Again, results are conflicting and study design can be criticized.

Having said all this, should you exercise? You bet! You'd better do it safely, however, because exercise can be harmful.

Exercising Safely

If you're voting age or greater, feel free to do all the walking you'd like. Do it at an easy pace. Don't attempt to work up a sweat. You're going too fast if you cannot comfortably breathe or talk while you walk.

This type of walking isn't intended to significantly elevate your heart rate or give you a workout. Before embarking on strenuous aerobic exercise, you'd better assess your cardiovascular risk factors. Doctors are very careful in not suggesting that you do anything vigorous without a thorough examination. That's because we don't want to be sued by you or, even worse, by your estate. So for starters, let's look at your risk.

1. Male sex
2. Cigarette smoker
3. Post-menopausal female
4. Taking the birth control pill especially if you're a smoker
5. History of high blood pressure whether treated or not
6. History of coronary heart disease (heart attack or angina)
7. Family history of coronary artery disease in a relative less than age 50

8. Elevated total blood cholesterol and/or elevated LDL cholesterol
9. History of sugar diabetes whether controlled by pills or insulin; history of sugar in your urine
10. Being more than 20 per cent above your "ideal" weight

As well, you'd best consider these other factors:

1. History of arthritis, joint or muscle disease
2. Pregnancy
3. Shortness of breath, asthma, emphysema, chronic bronchitis
4. History of dizziness, fainting spells, seizure disorder
5. Irregular or funny feeling heartbeats
6. History of pain, tightness or pressure in the chest that you haven't told your doctor about
7. Recent surgery or serious illness

If any of these 17 apply to you, or you can think of anything else that may prevent you from being physically active, you'd better see your doctor before embarking on any exercise program intended to increase your heart rate and hence your cardiovascular fitness. In many instances, your doctor will consider the visit unnecessary but, as the saying goes, it's better to be safe....

In other cases, after a physical examination and other appropriate tests such as a resting electrocardiogram and blood work, your doctor may suggest an exercise or stress electrocardiogram. Although in the minds of some doctors both tests are equivalent, they are different.

Testing Your Fitness

In a stress cardiogram you're hooked to a machine that is making tracings of the electrical impulses your heart is generating while you are either walking on a treadmill or pedalling on a stationary bike. The test is intended to see how long you can last and why you decided to quit, how your blood pressure responded to exercise, and whether or not there were certain changes present on the electrocardiogram that suggest coronary artery disease.

A stress EKG does have drawbacks, especially when symptomless people are being tested. Let's assume that 3 per cent of your adult neighbours have undetected coronary artery disease and that we run a stress EKG on everyone to find out who can safely exercise. Only a maximum of 85 per cent of those who actually have coronary heart disease will be picked up. That means of 100 people tested, 15 who appear healthy actually will have undetected heart disease. And since the test has only an 85 to 95 per cent chance of being able to recognize a normal person, 5 to 15 per cent of normal people will be called abnormal. When you consider the low incidence of a maximum of 3 per cent for asymptomatic heart disease in the general population, of 100 people with positive tests, only 13 of them will actually have coronary artery disease. The other 87 are what we call false positives. In actuality, they are normal. Thus in the population of people without known heart disease or symptoms, the predictive value of a stress cardiogram is not that great.

The imperfectness of stress EKGs is important for you to realize. You have to understand that a normal one does not guarantee that you won't suffer from coronary artery disease or that strenuous exercise is safe. And that an abnormal test, in a symptomless low-risk individual is more than likely a fault of the test, not of the testee's heart. Only further tests, like something called an exercise thallium scan perhaps, will tell.

A true fitness or exercise test involves measuring the maximum oxygen consumption of your body while you are doing a stress EKG. Aside from examining the EKG tracing for evidence of heart disease, another machine is continuously measuring the oxygen content of the air you breathe out. When you're at the point of exhaustion, the final measurement is called your maximum oxygen consumption, VO2 max for short. In addition the amount of carbon dioxide you breathe out and your respiratory rate can be measured.

These tests are based on the principle that the more physically active you are, the more oxygen your body burns and the faster your heart rate becomes. Thus by comparing your oxygen consumption to the general populations of your age and sex, you can get a good idea of how physically fit you are. Naturally, for someone who is about to embark on an exercise program, a test such as this is more useful than just a stress EKG. It will give you an idea of how you compare to everyone else and a baseline to determine your future progress against.

Sub-maximal stress cardiography and exercise testing should be done in a facility that is staffed by people trained to deal with cardiac emergencies. The test should not be done in fitness clubs, nor is it reasonable for you to ask your doctor for a letter indicating that you can partake in a vigorous exercise program or a fitness club-type fitness test. If you are going to have the test done, do it right, which unfortunately means in a facility that can afford the $60,000-plus in equipment that is required.

Choosing an Exercise Program

As far as the exercises themselves are concerned, you should have a program worked out for you by someone who knows what he or she is doing. For a good cardiovascular workout, you do not need to be a member of an expensive club. All you need is a pair of good shoes and somewhere to walk or jog. Swimming might be preferable to some people. Others may prefer a stationary bicycle, especially in the winter. If so, make your purchase from a reputable store where the salespeople know what they are selling and where you get a feeling that someone will be there to stand behind your purchase if there are problems. Try out the bicycles that are available. Consider a recumbent bike (one with a seat that has a back on it). These are very comfortable, especially if you have a history of a bad back, and they are quiet if you want to watch TV or listen to the stereo.

An exercise program that does not involve some warm-up and cool-down stretches has not been designed by anyone who knows what he or she is doing. The warm-up is intended to ready your muscles, heart, lungs and other body systems for the impending workout. It should take from three to five minutes and might involve rotation and bending of the neck, lateral trunk bending, slow and easy toe touches, stretches done with a towel behind your shoulders, and push-ups in the standing position back and forth against a wall.

When you and your fitness consultant have chosen an aerobic program, you'll be taught how to take your pulse and to what range of heart rate your exercise program is supposed to raise your resting pulse. As a general rule, your maximum pulse rate is calculated by subtracting your age from 220. The range that you'll be expected to achieve will fall somewhere between 45 to 80 per cent of your predicted maximum.

For example, a 40-year-old man will have a maximum predicted pulse rate of 220 - 40 = 180, giving him a target pulse range during exercise of between 81 and 144. Most people will train in the 65 to

80 per cent of maximum range, which in this case works out to 117 and 144. For a positive effect on your level of fitness, you have to exercise within your recommended pulse range for either four 20-minute sessions or three 30-minute sessions per week. Doing more isn't necessary and may even be harmful (too much of virtually anything can be detrimental). Doing less likely won't improve your level of endurance, although according to some of the studies it may still benefit you with regard to heart attack risk.

Table 10.1 Approximate Calories Used By 70 kg Person

Activity	Calories Per Minute	Calories Per Hour
Running, 11.4 m.p.h.	21.6	1,300
Running, 5.7 m.p.h.	12.0	720
Racquetball, squash	11.6	700
Skiing, cross-country, 5 m.p.h.	11.6	700
Swimming, crawl, 50 yds. minute	10.8	648
Skiing, downhill	10.0	600
Climbing stairs	9.8	590
Tennis, singles	9.0	540
Aerobic dancing, vigorous	8.5	510
Curling	8.0	480
Cycling, 10 m.p.h.	7.5	450
Gardening, weeding	5.6	336
Calisthenics	5.0	300
Swimming, crawl, 20 yds. minute	4.9	294
Walking, 3.5. m.p.h.	4.8	290
Aerobic dancing, mild	4.1	246
Bowling	4.0	240
Office work	2.4	145
Sleeping	1.1	70

A Cool-Down is Imperative

When you are done, a cool-down period is essential. From a cardiovascular point of view this may be the most dangerous period. If you've been exercising in standing or sitting positions, much of your blood volume may be pooled below the level of your heart. That's because of gravity and because the blood supply to the massive musculature of your legs was increased during the exercise period. Should you decide to abruptly stop your exercise program, the pooling effect may rob your heart or brain of an adequate blood supply and that, as you can imagine, may result in trouble.

Slow down slowly. Runners can jog; joggers can walk; walkers can slow their pace, shorten strides and swing their arms less. Stationary bicyclists can gradually release the tension and pedal more slowly. Swimmers should reduce their pace and stroke. Regardless of your choice of exercise, the cool-down should take five to ten minutes.

One final thing; don't take a sauna, whirlpool, steam bath or hot shower immediately after you exercise. All these activities lead to pooling of blood and they can accentuate the effects of the exercise itself. Cool down adequately first, and if you have a history of heart disease check with your doctor before engaging in any of these artificial sweatboxes.

Some exercise programs set up by professionals may contain an anaerobic phase. These include exercises in which our muscles require more oxygen than our systems can supply. Remarkably, to compensate, the muscles switch to a different energy-burning system that doesn't require oxygen, at least not initially. Examples of anaerobic exercise include sprinting and swimming under water. As a novice athlete, you should not be building up oxygen deficits by partaking in anaerobic exercise. As you can appreciate, it can be dangerous.

Personality and Your Heart

We can't say with certainty that your personality has anything to do with your cholesterol levels. But according to a report published 30 years ago, those intense people with what came to be called Type A personalities, were seven times more likely to suffer from heart disease than those with relaxed Type B behaviour.

That report came about 10 years after the "coronary-prone personality" was first described in some detail. And almost 40 years before that description, Sir William Osler, the father of modern medicine, had suggested that the psyche was a factor in the development of angina, the chest pain caused by inadequate blood flow through the heart's arteries, and of heart attack.

What is Type A behaviour? Perhaps a quote from one of the originators of the term, Dr. Meyer Friedman, would be appropriate. The co-author of *Type A Behaviour and Your Heart* described it as "a characteristic action-emotion complex, which is exhibited by those individuals who are engaged in a relatively chronic struggle to obtain an unlimited number of things from their environment in the shortest period of time and, if necessary, against the opposing forces of other things or persons in the same environment."

A Personal Catalogue

The author of this book, himself a Type A, once wrote a more down-to-earth summary: "To Type B's we usually appear overly alert, consumed by urgency, aggressive, and explosive in our speech. We work long hours, rarely take vacations, and are obsessive-compulsive about what we do. We grab authority, automatically seize responsibility, and are reluctant to share either. We tend to neglect ourselves; when we have problems, be they emotional or physical, we prefer to ignore them. We suffer from periodic depressions, which most of us don't recognize. Doing things slowly, or doing one thing at a time, is frustrating for us. We work quickly and have little or no patience with those who don't or won't keep up. Since we often have three, four or maybe even a dozen things on the go at once, we learn to juggle. Working to deadlines is an every day, if not every hour, reality."

Looking at a Type A, you might see tense facial muscles and, perhaps, sweating from the forehead or upper lip. Their postures may be rigid, and there may be forceful or restless movements of hands, fingers, fists, arms or legs. They tend to perch on the edge of their seats, seeming about to leap. In fact, it was Dr. Friedman's upholsterer who first noted the key link between cardiology and behaviour. When asked to re-do the doctor's office chairs, he remarked that the fabric was especially worn on the front edges.

Type A's also tend to be straightforward and opinionated. They get angry and hostile if you disagree with them or are incapable of understanding the "right" point of view. And they don't like to wait for anything, ever. They suffer from "hurry sickness," and usually have a spouse who is forever telling them to slow down.

In short, Type A's are impatient, competitive stress-seekers. Type B's are unhurried, easygoing stress-avoiders. These are the extremes, of course. Many people fall somewhere between, or move from one extreme to the other in differing circumstances.

The Association with Heart Disease

Although Type A's are hard-driving and aggressive, a surprising survey once found that more major U.S. corporations were headed by slow and steady B's. This sort of result doesn't necessarily mean that Type A's don't succeed; they're often both happy and satisfied with life. And their super-achiever tendencies can work to their benefit in unexpected ways.

For example, one study recently claimed that patients with A personalities had a lesser risk and lower death rate 12 years after their first heart attack. It was thought that only after such a threat to their lives did they direct their compulsive natures and intense drives for achievement toward changing their lifestyles and complying with medical therapy.

But when all the studies and medical opinions are considered, the association between heart disease and Type A behaviour isn't clear-cut. That's understandable; study design is part of the difficulty in all risk-factor research. It can always be criticized. Nor should we expect that there is a simple relationship between Type A and heart disease. If the Type A group is ever broken up into subgroups, we may well find that some groups are far more likely to have heart attacks than others. Some subgroups may turn out to have a below-average risk.

A similar sort of phenomenon was found with cholesterol. A high total cholesterol reading increases the risk of heart disease. LDL and HDL cholesterols are subgroups of total cholesterol, and it was discovered that if the LDL is up, the risk is even higher; but if the HDL is high, the risk of heart disease is lower.

Some preliminary research on Type A seems to indicate that anger and hostility are the elements most highly correlated with coronary artery disease. In addition, those who tend to hold their anger in may be doing their coronary arteries a disservice.

Given that heart disease causes about half the deaths in the western world, you might think that efforts are being made to identify those with Type A personalities - especially when some specialists consider this to be as important a risk factor as hypertension, smoking and elevated cholesterol. Well, there may be a Type A Behaviour Clinic somewhere in Canada; there may be doctors who specialize in converting A's to B's. But if there are, they're verging on the invisible.

Even though a review of the scientific literature on personality and heart disease makes it clear that some relationship exists, exactly what the relationship is and how to diagnose it are not clear. We can only hope that this situation improves soon. After all, the relationship was first suspected many decades ago, and identifying and modifying risk factors is the very foundation of preventive medicine.

What Can Happen To Type A's

Being a Type A can lead to many problems. Eventually, the frantic juggling of "priorities" becomes unproductive. Burn-out may arrive, with its fatigue, withdrawal, cynicism, forgetfulness and concentration difficulties. It may come before Type A's realize that their struggle with the world isn't worth the price. The price, of course, is also paid by family, friends, colleagues and associates.

What's unfortunate is that many Type A's don't realize just how high the price is until after they've had their first heart attack. More unfortunate are the Type A's who never realize it because they don't survive their first heart attack. Most fortunate are those who know they're Type A's and make some effort to change before something catastrophic occurs.

How to make that change is a large subject beyond the scope of this book. If you're a Type A, discuss it with your doctor, who may refer you to a psychologist, psychiatrist or other counsellor for help in learning how to be more of a Type B. Do it now - you want to be sure tomorrow comes.

Other Types of Stress

Although there is no certain relationship between stress and elevated cholesterol, several studies have shown that long-standing unpleasant emotions appear to be related to the development of coronary heart disease. These negative emotional states include anxiety, depression, anger, and dissatisfaction with life in general. The connection may be a result of increased activity in the autonomic nervous system or an increase in the fatty acid blood levels. Or it may be a result of the overeating, excess smoking and other compensations many people use in an attempt to deaden emotional pain.

There's little question that uncertainty and the fear of physical or psychological harm can affect our blood pressures. Hypertension is two to four times more prevalent in air traffic controllers, who spend their working lives facing the possibility of unexpected developments and tragic accidents.

Studies linking stress in general to heart disease in particular are few and far between. However, one well known study links life changes - both happy and unhappy - to an increased chance of illness or death from all causes, including heart attack. This doesn't mean that change is a bad thing, but rather that an accumulation of many changes in a short period of time may make us more susceptible to physical or emotional problems.

This shouldn't come as a great surprise; common sense would tell us that anyone going through change after change is under a lot of stress. One person may suffer only negative changes: being fired, divorced, injured, bereaved and bankrupted in the space of a year, for an actual example. Someone else may go through only positive changes: moving into a new home, getting married and having a baby, starting another career or job, winning a lottery, and taking the vacation of a lifetime.

But good or bad, when changes like these follow each other too quickly, we're in for an overload of stress. And if we have no control over the changes, or haven't learned coping strategies, we may be in for trouble down the road. A lack of satisfying relationships, social and family ties may be risk factors as well.

How to Manage Stress

A certain amount of stress is good for us. It keeps us on our toes and makes us perform at our best. Too little stress can leave us apathetic, irritable, unmotivated, bored - and boring. Too much, of course, can make us ill, age us before our time, and even kill us.

Whatever the cause, symptoms of a stress overload include being unable to sleep when you want to or should, fuzzy thinking and indecisiveness (it takes twice as long to do everything), poor memory, withdrawal and remoteness, an increase in or loss of appetite, excessive drinking, and the inability to keep things in perspective. Big things may make no impression on you at all, while small things cause you to overreact.

Keeping a balance in this case is more difficult than balancing one's diet, although adopting good eating habits will certainly help. So will a consistent exercise program that you like and can stay with. Depending on the situation, you may also need to do several or more of the following:

- Take relaxation lessons and try to sleep regular hours.
- Stop smoking and cut your alcohol and caffeine intake.
- Revive any family or social relationships you've let wither away.
- Vary your stresses by, say, interrupting your work with some vigorous exercise.
- See a marital or family therapist.
- Find a new boss or career or more workable situation.
- Take assertiveness-training classes.
- List your goals in life and decide if you really need to reach all of them.
- Insist that others involved in the situation share the stress load.
- Take time for yourself; give yourself some perks.
- Join a self-help group that offers mutual support for those with your particular concern, and read all you can on the subject.
- If no such group exists (for workaholics, say), start one yourself. Several Canadian cities have self-help resource centres to help you do this; most other cities have social agencies that will be glad to offer assistance.

This is hardly the definitive list of strategies for coping with stress, but it's a beginning. Making a list is the easy part. If you then decide to do nothing about your situation, you're setting yourself up to be a victim. You'll be at the mercy of whatever part of your body or your mind the stress chooses to attack.

Summary

1. Most weight problems are not related to hormonal problems, but they may be caused by behavioural disorders.
2. There is enough circumstantial evidence to suggest that regular aerobic exercise is good for your heart, lungs and your well being.
3. To be safe, check with your doctor before you begin exercising, and have your program designed by an expert.

4. While certain aspects of Type A behaviour seem to be related to coronary artery disease, the behaviour can be modified before it's too late.
5. Stress is especially dangerous to our health when we haven't learned how to handle it.

11

Drug Treatment

Under most circumstances, drugs aren't prescribed until a patient with elevated lipid levels has tried exercise and a lipid-lowering diet for a minimum of six months. And once drug treatment is begun, doctors always recommend that the patient continue his or her diet and exercise program.

Other patients simply don't seem to care about their health. Even after suffering a heart attack, some continue to smoke and won't watch what they eat. While purists might argue that people who won't help themselves don't deserve treatment, ethically they should be given the option of taking drugs to reduce their lipid levels.

When the decision to prescribe medication has been made, it is no longer enough for a doctor to hand you a prescription with the instructions: "Take this. I'll see you in three months." Drugs are expensive, and they can be harmful. You should be told how the drug works, what the side effects are, and what evidence exists proving that the drug will have other beneficial effects beyond the lowering of blood lipids. Many of the drugs available do this very well but have not as yet been shown to be associated with a reduction in heart disease or death.

The upcoming review of medications currently available

shouldn't be treated as gospel. Because some of the drugs are new on the market, those most prescribed today (drugs of choice) may be totally obsolete by the time you read this book. To make sure you get the latest information, discuss your prescription with your doctor or, if that isn't possible, with your pharmacist. If neither wants to answer your questions, find ones who will.

Bile Acid Sequestrants

The drugs of choice at the moment for those with elevated LDL cholesterol levels are the bile acid sequestrants. The generic names for the two available are cholestyramine and colestipol; their brand names are Questran and Colestid. To help you understand how they work, here's a brief review of how bile works.

A detergent used to help us absorb fat, bile comes from the liver and is stored in the gall-bladder until we eat a meal containing fat. Then a hormone causes the gall-bladder to contract, squeezing the bile and its cholesterol-containing bile acids out into the bile duct and the first part of the small intestine. There, bile mixes with semi-digested food and aids in fat absorption. Some bile acids are themselves reabsorbed into the bloodstream, where they are ferried off to the liver along with the fat. Once in the liver, they begin their journey all over again. Since the bile acids are circulated from liver to intestine to liver, the process is called the enterohepatic circulation.

Bile acid sequestrants attach to the acids in the intestine and prevent some of them from being absorbed back into the body. In essence, they disrupt the enterohepatic circulation. Since fewer bile acids are returned to the liver, it's forced to produce more to make up for the loss. This increased production - and it may increase up to ten times - results in the liver using up cholesterol to manufacture bile acids.

The liver produces more cholesterol but also removes more LDL from the blood. As a result, LDL levels fall by 20 to 35 per cent. Total cholesterol may fall by 15 to 20 per cent, with HDL increasing by 2 to 5 per cent. The bile acids bound to the sequestrant are excreted from the body with the stools.

Both drugs come in powder form; four grams of cholestyramine is equivalent to five grams of colestipol. (While purchasing them in bulk is cheaper than buying individual packets, at present only cholestyramine is available in bulk in Canada.) They're mixed with water, juice or other liquids and usually taken twice a day, 30 minutes before or after your two largest meals. Some doctors suggest beginning with one scoop or package before or after only the evening meal for the first week. That's because some patients experience bloating or nausea that might be worse if they began with a higher dose. Most become accustomed to the drug quite quickly, however, and these bothersome side effects tend to go away by themselves.

You'll find that these drugs don't dissolve entirely in the liquid; no matter what you mix them with, you'll be drinking small particles. For this reason, some people mix their drinks in a blender to improve consistency and palatability. After mixing, the drink should be allowed to sit for a few minutes to ensure that all the particles have been wetted. Then just give it a stir and drink up.

After a month of treatment, your blood lipids should be measured. If they're still elevated, the dose can be increased to up to six packs or scoops per day. Since there is no emergency, increasing the dose by one package or scoop per month is reasonable.

Side Effects of Bile Acid Sequestrants

After temporary bloating and nausea, the next most common side effect is constipation. Increasing your fluid intake might help, as might eating more fibre, which you should be doing anyway. Sometimes, it may be necessary to take a stool softener.

Since these drugs aren't absorbed by your body, they produce no serious internal side effects. They've been on the market for quite some time, and it's pretty well accepted that they are safe for prolonged use. In fact, both are safe even for children and women of childbearing potential. Most important, they have been proven effective in preventing coronary artery disease.

However, the bile acid sequestrants may delay or prevent the absorption of such drugs as digitoxin, thyroxin, phonobarbital, tetracycline, phenylbutazone, and anticoagulants like coumadin/ warfarin. So if you are taking these or any other medications, do so at least one hour before or four hours after you take the sequestrant.

Niacin (Nicotinic Acid or Vitamin B-3)

One of the B-complex vitamins, nicotinic acid was isolated from tobacco way back in 1867. Many years later, doctors realized that lack of it in the body caused a vitamin-deficiency disease called pellagra. The name was changed to niacin to avoid confusion between nicotinic acid and nicotine.

Pellagra is characterized by the four Ds: dermatitis (skin rash), diarrhea, depression and death. We usually get the niacin we need through food or through the body's conversion of one of the protein building blocks, the amino acid called tryptophan. It takes 60 mg of tryptophan for our bodies to manufacture 1 mg of niacin. Good dietary sources of both include milk, eggs, meat, poultry, fish and other protein foods, whole grain and enriched breads, cereals and nuts.

To maintain health and prevent pellagra the average woman requires 13 mg of niacin per day, the average man 18. But to lower elevated levels of VLDL and LDL takes from 1000 to 7000 mg (1 to 7 grams) per day. Since the niacin is being used in mega-doses to treat a disease rather than a vitamin deficiency, it is now classified as a drug. While you can still buy it over the counter without a prescription, *no one* should take lipid-lowering doses of niacin without first clearing it with a doctor. Don't confuse it with nicotinamide or buy it in combination with other B-complex vitamins, none of which will lower lipids. If your doctor has told you to take niacin for your lipid problem, you are taking a drug, not a vitamin supplement. It must be treated with respect and the doses recommended by your doctor shouldn't be exceeded.

Niacin is a very powerful lipid-lowering drug. Total cholesterol may drop 20 per cent, LDL 25 per cent and triglycerides more than 40 per cent. HDL may rise by 20 percent, which may be particularly significant. Some people who have heart attacks have relatively normal total cholesterols but low HDLs. Like the bile acid sequestrants, niacin has been shown to prevent heart disease and heart attack-related death. It probably lowers lipids by decreasing fatty acid flux from cells and by reducing the production of lipoproteins in the liver.

Side Effects of Niacin

Unfortunately, niacin isn't the perfect drug. Side effects are so common that up to 40 per cent of those on the drug stop taking it. They just can't tolerate doses high enough to lower their lipids and increase HDLs.

The most common side effect is flushing of the skin. Alcohol, caffeine (coffee, tea, chocolate, cola drinks) and spicy foods should be avoided because they may accentuate the flushing. Taking the niacin with meals may help, too. (A slow-release preparation not available in Canada may reduce the flushing, but it can increase liver and gut-related side effects and doesn't lower lipids as effectively.) Taking half an adult size ASA 30 minutes before the niacin may also help prevent flushing.

Most doctors start their patients on niacin slowly. Some prefer to start with 100 mg tablets, three times per day for the first week. Then the blood is checked to see what effects there have been on lipids, liver function and uric acid levels, and the dose is increased as necessary. Other doctors begin with 500 mg taken with dinner for three days. If side effects aren't too bad, 500 mg is then added with lunch for the next three days. If that is tolerated, another 500 mg is added with breakfast. Blood tests can be done and doses adjusted accordingly.

After about two weeks at a particular dose level, the flushing should become tolerable. However, if you miss taking your niacin for even a couple of days, the flushing will be back when you start again. With doses above 2000 mg (2 grams) per day, there may be irritation of the liver, which can be picked up by a blood test to measure liver enzymes. Mild elevations of uric acid could theoretically cause an attack of gout or very rarely a uric acid kidney stone. Rarely, too, blood sugar levels may become elevated.

Blurred vision and other visual disturbances are rare, but if they occur a doctor should be consulted immediately and the niacin discontinued permanently. Heartburn could be another reason to see a doctor; niacin can be associated with recurrence of peptic ulcers.

In short, niacin could be dangerous in high doses. Everyone taking it should receive periodic medical monitoring, blood tests included.

Lovastatin (Mevacor)

A relatively new drug, lovastatin is well tolerated by about 98 per cent of the population. And it has the advantage that many patients need take it only once a day. It lowers cholesterol by 18 to 34 per cent, LDL by 19 to 39 per cent, and increases HDL 3 to 13 per cent. Hence, like niacin, it does all the right things to your lipids.

Lovastatin works by inhibiting the enzyme that controls the speed of the slowest step in the liver's cholesterol production plant.

In addition, it appears to promote the destruction of LDL cholesterol in the liver. The starting and usual maintenance dose of 20 mg is taken with the evening meal. If the dose has to be increased, the maximum is 80 mg per day, half of which may be taken with breakfast. The incidence of unpleasant side effects is considerably less than with niacin or cholystyramine and, being a pill, lovastatin doesn't taste unpleasant like the powders. Based on all these factors, it may well become the most popular cholesterol-lowering drug.

Side Effects of Lovastatin

What might limit lovastatin's popularity is added clinical experience. Because it's a fairly new medication, most of the side-effect information is based on studies of six years or less. We need to know more about any long-term side effects. This data will come as those who have been on the drug since the early studies continue to take it.

In addition, lovastatin has not been shown to reduce the incidence of arteriosclerosis, coronary artery disease, heart attack or related death. In theory, anything that decreases "bad" cholesterol and increases the "good" HDL cholesterol should lower one's chances of developing these problems. As far as lovastatin is concerned, however, that has not yet been proven in a study. While a purist might argue that on this basis cholystyramine and niacin are preferable, the purist doesn't have to personally tolerate the side effects of these drugs.

Among those who should not take lovastatin are women who may become pregnant, and anyone who is on such medications as cyclosporine, corticosteroids or anti-coagulants. In addition, those taking gemfibrozil (Lopid) and lipid-lowering doses of niacin (nicotinic acid) should not be simultaneously taking lovastatin, since drug interactions may occur. The drug should also not be taken by people suffering from liver disease.

Possible side effects of lovastatin include aching muscles, muscle cramping, tiredness, weakness, fever or blurred vision. Other side effects may come and go occasionally, including abdominal pain, constipation, diarrhea, nausea, headache, dizziness and skin rashes.

If you are prescribed lovastatin, you should receive and read the patient information sheet prepared by its manufacturer, then discuss the contents with your doctor. You must have regular medical follow-ups and periodic blood tests. You should also see an eye doctor before beginning the drug, and annually thereafter.

Probucol (Lorelco)

Although it's known that probucol lowers total and LDL-cholesterol in human beings, how it does this just isn't known. From tests on rabbits, it has been suggested that the drug makes changes to the LDL cholesterol complex, resulting in it being cleared from the blood at a quicker rate. In some people probucol lowers total cholesterol in the 15 to 20 per cent range while at the same time lowering LDL up to 20 per cent. In other people, however, its cholesterol-lowering effects are not all that marked.

Of concern is the fact that probucol decreases the good HDL cholesterol, but the significance of this effect is not clear. When this drug is prescribed, periodic monitoring of total, HDL and LDL cholesterol levels would be wise. If the lowering effect on LDL is only temporary, discontinuing the medication should be considered, especially if it has lowered HDL levels significantly. No matter how your elevated lipids are treated, periodic monitoring and competent medical assessment are required.

Side Effects of Probucol

The usual dose is 500 mg a day. Side effects are usually minimal and include diarrhea, gas, abdominal pain and nausea. You should have an electrocardiograph (EKG) run prior to taking this medication, and perhaps a follow-up one after you've been on it for a while. Although probucol causes changes in the cardiograph of some people, such changes have not been associated with any problems. Nonetheless, those with certain abnormalities on their EKG shouldn't take this medication.

Once in your system, probucol is stored in your fat cells. The cholesterol-lowering effect may continue for many weeks after you stop taking it, as the drug stored in your fat re-enters the bloodstream. Hence, this is not a drug of preference if you're a woman of child-bearing age, unless you are using an effective form of birth control.

D-thyroxine (Choloxin)

The naturally occurring thyroid hormone is L-thyroxine. D-thyroxine might be called a mirror image. It can lower cholesterol by about 20 per cent. It lowers LDL by stimulating receptors in the liver, which leads to increased removal of LDL from the blood, but it does not affect triglycerides or HDL.

The usual dose is 1 to 2 mg daily for one month, at which point your lipid levels are measured. If the desired effect hasn't been achieved, the dose can be increased by 1 to 2 mg per month up to a maximum of 8 mg per day. In high doses, D-thyroxine may aggravate or bring on the chest pain symptoms of angina. Thus it is not recommended for anyone with diagnosed coronary artery disease or for older patients who may have undiagnosed heart disease.

Although not nearly as powerful in its hormonal action as L-thyroxine, this drug still has some effect. And that may cause such side effects as sweating, nervousness, tremor, sleeping problems and rapid heart rate. For this reason, it is usually prescribed only for young, otherwise healthy, people with elevated cholesterols. And then only after diet, exercise and some of the other drugs described here have not controlled the problem.

Clofibrate (Atromid-S)

In a World Health Organization study, the use of clofibrate resulted in fewer non-fatal heart attacks. But it did not seem to prevent deaths caused by heart attack, and there was an increased rate in deaths from other causes. Some were from cancer; others from gallstone complications. (Clofibrate is known to increase the risk of developing gallstones.)

The major action of this drug is on triglycerides. It can decrease levels by 40 per cent. It lowers VLDL (very low density lipoprotein) within two to five days. In most cases there is also a fall in total cholesterol and LDL. However, in some the LDL does not change significantly, and in others it increases. All in all, a drug to consider only if triglyceride levels are very high and other therapies have failed.

Gemfibrozil (Lopid)

Using clofibrate as a model, chemists created some 8,700 other compounds and tested them for their lipid-lowering properties. Gemfibrozil, created in 1968, turned out to be the most effective and safest of the lot.

Because it acts predominantly on the triglyceride-rich VLDL's, this is not a drug of first choice for anyone whose primary problem is elevated cholesterol or LDL. It can increase LDL in some people with high triglycerides so it is very important that LDL levels be monitored on a regular basis. If the LDL does go up, adding one of the bile acid sequestrant drugs may bring it back down.

Table 11.1 Effect of Drugs on Blood Lipids[1]

Drug	Dosage	HDL	Triglycerides
Cholestyramine (Questran)	12-24 g	No effect or increases	No effect or increases
Colestipol (Colestid)	15-30 g	No effect or increases	No effect or increases
Niacin or nicotinic acid	1.5-6.0 g	Increases	Lowers
Lovastatin (Mevacor)	20-80 mg	No effect or increases	No effect or lowers
Probucol (Lorelco)	500-1000 mg	Lowers	No effect
D-thyroxine (Choloxin)	2-6 mg	No effect	No effect
Clofibrate (Atromid-S)	1-2 g	No effect or increases	Lowers
Gemfibrozil (Lopid)	600-1200 mg	Increases	Lowers

[1] All eight of these drugs lower total and LDL-cholesterol

Gemfibrozil does have the advantage of increasing levels of good HDL in most of those taking it, however.

Side effects include mild nausea, diarrhea and stomach upset in about 5 per cent of patients. There may be muscle aches, skin rashes or an increased chance of developing gallstones. An increase in blood sugar is a rare side effect, but it must be considered in the case of diabetics.

On the up side, the so-called Helsinki study found that gemfibrozil had fewer side effects than the bile acid sequestrants, nicotinic acid or clofibrate. And most important, it was shown to effectively reduce the incidence of coronary heart disease. Clearly, this drug has proven benefits. Just as clearly, it is not a good drug for everyone.

Summary

Although we have a number of effective lipid-lowering drugs, it's obvious that the perfect medication has not yet been developed. Each of the drugs outlined has good and not-so-good characteristics. All the drugs affect blood lipids (see Table 11.1), but cholestyramine, colestipol, nicotinic acid and gemfibrozil have been shown to reduce the incidence of both fatal and non-fatal heart attacks. There is even evidence that some of these drugs can slow the rate of atherosclerosis and perhaps even reverse existing disease in the coronary arteries.

In theory, though, fewer than 5 per cent of those with hyperlipidemia should require drugs. In practice, provincial health plans rarely pay for professional diet counselling unless it is done in a clinic or hospital setting. Nor is there adequate teaching of nutrition at the elementary, high school or university level, and that includes medical schools.

Even so, no responsible physician should immediately write a prescription for a lipid-lowering medication. No intelligent patient should be taking drugs without first having received information on diet and exercise therapy. Resources are in short supply, but having an elevated cholesterol does entitle you to an appointment with a nutritionist who has an interest in lipid problems.

12

The Bottom Line

We've been asking you to make some significant changes in your lifestyle. But you want some evidence that there *is* a relationship between blood cholesterol and heart disease. As an intelligent person, you'll want scientific proof from various sources and from different types of studies. With some reservations you'll accept animal studies, but you'll require proof from human experiments. Well, here it is.

We won't get into the ethics of animal experimentation; we'll just acknowledge the fact that some is done when the experiments are too risky to attempt on human beings.

Not surprisingly monkeys make good experimental subjects. Some of our tree-dwelling brethren develop atherosclerotic plaques and thickenings very similar to ours. If one feeds rhesus monkeys a typical North American diet high in fat, protein and sugars, they develop elevated blood cholesterols and severe atherosclerosis. However, when fed a more prudent diet lower in fat, saturated fat and cholesterol, atherosclerosis is less frequent and not as severe.

While few would be proud that science can induce disease in animals, there may be satisfaction in knowing that the disease *can* be reversed significantly after a year or so on a prudent diet.

Epidemiologic Studies

Surveys that compare countries, people, regions or groups of similar people living in different places are epidemiologic studies. In essence, they compare one clearly defined population to another defined population. When one major study compared what quantities of foods different countries consumed and the causes of death of their inhabitants, it was found that the higher the per-person caloric intake, total fat, saturated fat, cholesterol, protein and sugars, the higher the country's incidence of death caused by coronary artery disease. Another study compared arteries and diets by examining autopsy results. The conclusion from 23,000 autopsies done in 12 countries: there is a direct relationship between total dietary fat consumption and the amount of atherosclerosis. The greater the fat intake, the more plaque in the arteries.

A third survey asked some 12,000 men in seven countries - Yugoslavia, the U.S., the Netherlands, Japan, Italy, Greece and Finland - about their diets and other heart disease risk factors. The losers were Finland and the U.S., where the incidence of coronary artery disease was the highest. The winners were Japan and three areas in Greece, where the incidence was low. Saturated fat intakes and cholesterol levels were highest where coronary artery disease was most common.

But how do we know there isn't something other than diet that results in the low incidence of heart disease in Japan? To answer that question, people of Japanese native origin living in Japan, Honolulu and San Francisco were compared. And it was found that someone of Japanese ancestry was more likely to die of a heart attack in San Francisco than in Honolulu, although the likelihood was still higher in Honolulu than in Japan. Saturated fat intake in Japan was half what it was in San Francisco. Average body weight in Japan was 55 kg; in San Francisco, 66 kg. Cholesterol levels in San Francisco were 21 per cent higher than in Japan. In each factor, Honolulu with its intermediate death rate fell between San Francisco and Japan. Proof that it's not simply being Japanese that is responsible for a lower incidence of heart disease. What seems to be important is the lower intake of saturated fat in the native Japanese diet.

People within the same country who have different dietary habits have also been compared. True vegetarians have a diet low in saturated fat and devoid of cholesterol. Lacto-ovo vegetarians allow themselves eggs and dairy products, both of which contain cholesterol, and their saturated fat intakes are higher. By now, we shouldn't be astounded by the fact that strict vegetarians have lower cholesterol levels and less heart disease than lacto-ovo vegetarians. (But the latter still have healthier hearts than those who eat meat.)

Prospective Studies

Although time-consuming and very expensive, prospective studies are the cleanest type. Ideally, a population of similar people is separated into groups, followed for a number of years, then compared.

Probably the most famous of all prospective studies was the Lipid Research Clinics Coronary Primary Prevention Trial. Carried out in 12 cities across North America, including two in Canada, more than 300,000 men were screened to recruit the 3,806 who ultimately took part. Each middle-aged man had to appear healthy and have a total cholesterol over 265 mg/dl (6.85 mmol/L) and an LDL greater than 170 mg/dl (4.39 mmol/L). After being divided into two groups taking into account other risk factors such as cigarette smoking, each group was put on a diet that lowered blood cholesterol by about 4 per cent. One group also received a placebo (inactive) medication while the other was given cholestyramine (see Chapter 11).

The group taking the drug had on average a blood cholesterol 9 per cent lower and LDL 12 per cent lower than the placebo group. The more the medication lowered a man's cholesterol, the less likely he was to suffer from a heart attack. On average, what the study showed was that for every 1 per cent drop in blood cholesterol over a period of years, there was about a 2 per cent drop in the risk of developing coronary artery disease. In addition to fewer heart attacks and coronary-related deaths, the drug group had fewer cases of angina and few cases of coronary artery bypass surgery.

The Oslo Study was designed to see what would happen to 1,232 middle-aged men with normal blood pressures if they stopped smoking and lowered their cholesterol levels. Two groups were studied over five years and, when all was done, a special intervention group had reduced its cholesterols by an average of 13 per cent. And there was a more than 40 per cent reduction in heart attacks and sudden death caused by heart disease. While very impressive, the results can't be attributed entirely to the lower cholesterol. Reduction or cessation of smoking likely played some role.

Diet and Reversal Studies

The Wadsworth Veterans Administration Hospital Study is an example of a diet trial study. Some of the 846 male participants, average age 65, had evidence of coronary artery disease. They were assigned on a random basis to either a control (normal diet) or an experimental (cholesterol-lowering diet) group. Basically the diets differed in the percentage of calories received from saturated versus polyunsaturated fats. After eight years of follow-up, heart attacks and associated deaths were 31 per cent less in those on a diet high in polyunsaturated fats.

What about studies to show that atherosclerosis, once established, can be reversed? In the U.S. National Heart, Lung and Blood Institute Type II Hyperlipidemia Trial, people with known coronary artery disease were treated with the drug cholestyramine and a cholesterol-lowering diet, then compared to similar people on the same diet taking placebo medication. In both groups after five years of study, a drop in the LDL cholesterol and an increase in the HDL correlated to less progression of arterial disease confirmed by angiograms (dye X-rays). In the Leiden Study, 39 men with coronary artery disease were studied with coronary angiograms, then put on a diet high in polyunsaturates and low in cholesterol (less than 100 mg). After two years, repeat angiograms showed no advancement of arterial disease in those able to maintain lower levels of total cholesterol and higher levels of HDL.

Finally, in the Cholesterol Lowering Atherosclerosis Study, 162 men who had undergone coronary bypass surgery were treated with diet or diet and a combination of drugs (colestipol and niacin). Unfortunately, in the non-drug group there was only a 4 per cent drop in total cholesterol, with a 5 per cent fall in LDL. In the diet-plus-drug group, however, the cholesterol fell some 26 per cent and the LDL went down 43 per cent. At the same time HDL increased and triglyceride levels toppled. The favorable lipid responses were associated with a reduced tendency for new atherosclerotic narrowing in both the grafted and natural arteries. And there was evidence to suggest that some of the plaque had regressed.

The Summing Up

On examining an aggregate of diet studies, there appears to be a trend suggesting that for every 1 per cent reduction in total cholesterol, there's a 1 to 1.5 per cent reduction in the risk of developing heart disease. Examination of an aggregate of drug trials puts the number closer to a 2 per cent reduction in risk for every 1 per cent drop in total cholesterol.

What We Now Know

1. Heart and blood-vessel diseases are major killers. Likely half of us will eventually die as a result of such cardiovascular problems. Eighty thousand deaths per year in Canada is as good an estimate as any.

2. The cost to Canadians for medical care and absenteeism resulting from cardiovascular disease is about $1.3 billion annually.

3. Cardiovascular disease has many contributing causes. Most of those who develop it, especially if they do so before they reach 55, have more than one risk factor.

4. It's unrealistic to think that modification of a single risk factor will cure heart disease. That's because major risk factors include a family history of heart disease, advancing age and being a male.

5. Other risk factors include tobacco smoking, elevated blood cholesterol, diabetes, high blood pressure, obesity, physical inactivity, and a stressful lifestyle. All can be modified or changed if you want to change them.

6. If you smoke and want to live longer, give up the habit. Of all these risk factors, smoking is the most likely to lead to your premature death.

7. If you don't know what your blood pressure is, you should have it checked. If it's high, have a sensible discussion with your doctor about the best way to get it back into the normal range.

When It Comes to Cholesterol ...

1. Heart and blood-vessel disease caused by deposits in the arteries or atherosclerosis is more common on this continent than in many other parts of the world.

2. Our diets are higher in total fat, saturated fat and cholesterol than those of people living in areas of the world where heart and blood-vessel disease occur less often.

3. The levels of total cholesterol and LDL in our blood are higher than those of people living in parts of the world where heart and blood-vessel disease are less common.

4. There is scientific evidence, particularly in relation to middle-aged men, supporting the theory that the higher one's blood cholesterol and LDL, the higher the risk of having heart and blood-vessel disease.

5. There is scientific evidence, particularly as it applies to middle-aged men, supporting the theory that the higher the blood level of one's HDLs, the lower one's risk of developing heart and blood-vessel disease.

6. There is scientific evidence to suggest that if a middle-aged man with a very high level of blood cholesterol reduces it by following a prudent diet and using certain medications, his chances of suffering from heart and blood-vessel disease decline.

7. There is no evidence to suggest that sticking to a prudent diet will in any way harm an otherwise healthy adult.

8. There are many drugs that will effectively lower cholesterol levels. However, there is no direct evidence to show that some of them will reduce heart or blood-vessel disease as a result, and we still don't know the long-term effects of many of them. As a result, lowering your blood cholesterol by altering your diet is preferable to taking medications.

9. It is very important to understand the basic facts about nutrition. Good health results from a balanced diet. Maintaining an ideal

weight will result only from balanced dieting. There is no such thing as bad food, bad fat, or bad anything in the way of nutrition. "Bad" and "good" are extremes; most things are somewhere in the middle. While you may have to limit your intake of certain foods to achieve an over-all balanced, prudent diet, few of us need to go to extremes.

10. If dietary modifications have not brought your cholesterol down to a safer level and drugs are prescribed, make sure you know the potential short- and long-term side effects and that you attend follow-up visits with your doctor on a periodic basis.

11. Increasing physical activity at the very least will make you feel better. It may also contribute to reaching or maintaining your ideal weight, lowering your total and LDL cholesterol, lowering your blood pressure, and raising your protective HDL cholesterol.

Test Your Knowledge

(Answers on next page)

TRUE or FALSE?

1. Heart disease can never be prevented or delayed.

2. If your relatives developed early coronary artery disease, you are at a greater risk of developing it yourself.

3. Signs of atherosclerosis are never found in infants and children.

4. The major determinant of blood cholesterol concentrations is the absolute intake of saturated fatty acids.

5. High-density lipoprotein (HDL) cholesterol protects our blood vessels from atherosclerosis.

6. Your total fat intake should be no more than 30 per cent of your day's calories.

7. Your fat intake should be divided equally among saturated, polyunsaturated and mono-unsaturated fats.

8. Complex carbohydrates raise cholesterol levels.

135

9. Oat bran and a number of fruits and vegetables have been reported to have a beneficial effect on cholesterol levels.

10. Stress and other lifestyle risk factors have no relationship to coronary artery disease.

11. High blood pressure, diabetes and obesity are risk factors for coronary artery disease.

12. Heart and blood-vessel disease caused by atherosclerosis is more common on this continent than in many other parts of the world.

13. There is evidence that the higher one's blood cholesterol and LDL, the higher one's risk of heart and blood-vessel disease.

14. Increasing physical activity may contribute to raising your protective HDL cholesterol.

15. More than anything else, smoking increases your risk of premature death.

Answers to
Test Your Knowledge

1. False.	2. True.	3. False.	4. True.	5. True.
6. True.	7. True.	8. False.	9. True.	10. False.
11. True.	12. True.	13. True.	14. True.	15. True.

APPENDIX 1

The Canadian Consensus Conference on Cholesterol

In March, 1988, a two-day conference was held in Ottawa. Its purpose was to come up with a national viewpoint on the prevention of heart and vascular disease by altering blood cholesterol and lipoprotein risk factors. A final report containing many recommendations was issued by a 12-person panel, whose members included a family doctor, biochemists, a pediatrician, nutritionists, medical specialists and a lawyer.

You have read about several of the Canadian Consensus Conference on Cholesterol recommendations in earlier sections of this book, but all of them have a potential impact on the cardiovascular health of Canadians. Here, then, is a summary, followed by some personal views.

Health Promotion: All levels of government, as well as voluntary agencies, should give high priority to information campaigns about all cardiovascular risk factors. These programs, said the panel, "should enlist all relevant sections of the economy, involve all health care disciplines and be allocated enough resources to be effective in reducing population risk."

Dietary Guidelines: Canadians should be advised to reduce their fat intake to about 30 per cent of total daily calories, with saturated fats accounting for 10 per cent or less (see also Diet Modification).

137

Role of Agriculture and Food Industry: It should be encouraged to produce healthy foods; restaurants, cafeterias and other caterers should be encouraged to offer meals low in fat and cholesterol; consumers should receive better information about nutrient content.

Population Goal: Public health programs should aim to achieve an average cholesterol level of 4.9 mmol/L (190 mg/dl) for Canadians as a whole.

Lipid and Lipoprotein Risk Factors: The panel felt that tests for total cholesterol, triglyceride and HDL cholesterol were the minimum required to determine lipid risk factors. (Laboratories routinely calculate LDL using a mathematical formula.)

Patients with Priorities for Testing: These include those with known heart disease, a family history of hyperlipidemia or early coronary artery disease, high blood pressure, diabetes, kidney failure and obesity, especially abdominal obesity. As resources permit, testing of more than just total cholesterol should be part of every adult's periodic health examinations, with priority given to those who have other risk factors.

Management of Hypercholesterolemia: These are the cholesterol level and treatment guidelines shown Table 3.1. The panel expected that working groups would be set up to establish more detailed guidelines.

Diet Modification: This, said the panel, remains the principal treatment for elevated blood fats. (See Chapters 6, 7, 8 and 9.) With fat at 30 per cent or less and protein at 10 to 15 per cent, the remainder of the day's intake should be provided by carbohydrates, particularly various forms of dietary fibre. We should try to get enough physical activity to "achieve and maintain" cardiovascular fitness, and balance that with just enough calories to stay at an acceptable body weight. Some patients will require diets with less than 30 per cent fat and under 300 mg of cholesterol; some may need to restrict alcohol, sugar or sodium intake as well.

Children, however, should not be put on a parent's diet. They need a varied diet that includes all the major food groups and a fat intake of 30 to 40 per cent, with calories adjusted to maintain a healthy weight.

Other Risk Factors: The adverse effects of cigarette smoking, high blood pressure, diabetes, obesity and a sedentary lifestyle should be publicized in health promotion programs for all Canadians.

Drug Therapy: This should be used only after "rigorous diet modification" for six months has failed, and "intensive" diet therapy should continue. In some cases where the lipid abnormality is profound or specific, it may be appropriate to start drug therapy along with dietary changes.

Laboratory Services and Educational Programs: The panel felt that to make its recommendations feasible, laboratory facilities had to be expanded to handle the volume of work, and upgraded as well. To "ensure accurate measurement" provincial and federal governments should "set analytical goals and take steps to improve and standardize assays through the establishment and funding of reference laboratories for lipids and lipoproteins." (The latter is now taking place.)

For physicians and other health care personnel, there should be national education programs on the diagnosis and treatment of people at risk. The provinces should take immediate steps to provide more dietitians, offer further education for those already in the field and, to cope with the present shortage, consider such innovative approaches as group dietary counselling and support groups. As well, we should think about having a national cholesterol education program in schools, workplaces and other community settings.

Research and Development Priorities: The panel concluded its report by pointing out that the need for research exists in every area relevant to cardiovascular disease - biomedical, clinical, nutritional, health services, public health, social and behavioural aspects.

The Consensus Conference was the first gathering to emphasize to the public, health care professionals and industry the importance of elevated cholesterol as a cardiovascular risk factor, and a large number of experts made presentations on the subject. While the final report was a good beginning, some Canadian health care professionals felt it didn't provide them with enough specific information. It couldn't, because medical science just doesn't know enough to allow an official body to come out with blanket recommendations.

Nevertheless, I am about to make some suggestions on how the panel's recommendations might be implemented. If you agree with my views, remember that as a taxpayer, voter, consumer, customer, employee, employer, parent or concerned patient, you do have the right to push for change where you feel it is necessary.

Health Promotion

There is no question that prevention works. Although overwhelming scientific evidence shows a relationship between lifestyle, environment and the development of heart disease, there is also enormous evidence that modifications we make ourselves can result in healthier hearts. Those who are free of heart disease can delay or prevent its development; those who have atherosclerosis, angina and similar problems, or who've had a heart attack or stroke, may prevent further disease from developing. In some cases, we can even reverse disease that is already established.

When we think, teach and practise prevention, however, we should keep in mind that it's a many-splendoured and highly rewarding endeavour only if we incorporate as much of it as possible into our lives. While modifying one risk factor like high cholesterol with diet is great, the effect becomes far greater when combined with giving up smoking; greater still when we attain an ideal weight and exercise regularly. Not only that, these positive changes may prevent other diseases, such as some forms of cancer.

That's why preventive information must get out to the public from all levels of government as well as voluntary agencies, as the Consensus panel recommends. Boards of education, for example, have made an impact with their anti-smoking campaigns: children in elementary school are now among Canada's strongest proponents of a smoke-free environment. It would be a relatively simple matter to teach them that fatty foods and simple sugars are less desirable nutrients than other foods.

Role of Agriculture and Food Industry

In my opinion, cafeterias under any form of public control (such as those in schools, hospitals, government buildings and airports) should have to guarantee as part of their lease agreements that they will provide a choice of nutritious food. In some of these cafeterias, it's impossible to stick to a healthy diet; good food choices simply don't exist. Where they do, the food is often presented in such an unappetizing way that few would dare to choose it.

Cafeterias in the private sector must be urged to offer healthy food that adheres to Canada's Food Guide and other guidelines suggested by the Consensus panel. Employers in both the public and private sectors should be promoting good health for both their own and their employees' benefit; unions and similar organizations could cooperate both spiritually and financially.

Certainly the food industry should be lobbied to develop and promote foods that give us protection against heart disease, cancer and other forms of illness. Government might even be persuaded to limit the fat content of some foods, ban the use of certain types of fats, and legislate more prominent labelling of food.

I'd like to see every restaurant, fast food outlet, cafeteria, food retailer, wholesaler and manufacturer list the contents and nutritional composition of every product they offer to the public. At present, some manufacturers, retailers and restaurateurs seem to have no idea what's in the foodstuffs they sell. Others will supply information if it's requested by phone or mail but don't display that information at point of sale. Not only does this make it difficult for us to make prudent choices, it's also dangerous for those with food allergies and sensitivities.

My suggestion is not an impossible dream. The federal and provincial governments cooperated with labour and management in the formation of WHIMIS (workplace hazardous information) to ensure that anyone who's interested can determine the potential hazards of manufactured goods. It's not unreasonable for us to expect the same approach for the food we put in our mouths. Voluntary agencies like those that sponsored the Consensus Conference, and/or such public agencies as Health and Welfare Canada, might even consider endorsing certain foods that comply with appropriate guidelines.

You and I have the power to shape, if not dictate, public policy. It's time we began to lobby all levels of government, private sector employers, unions, school boards and restaurant chains for help in our quest for better health generally and better cholesterol levels specifically.

Population Goal

While the panel felt the mean or average cholesterol value for Canadians should be 4.9 mmol/L (190 mg/dl), it acknowledged that this was a long-term goal. Cholesterol levels are dependent on age, sex and hormone status (some birth control pills and hormones taken in the menopause can affect levels), but in general the lower one's blood cholesterol, the lower the risk of developing coronary artery disease. The ideal combination is a high level of HDL, with relatively low levels of total cholesterol and LDL, as shown below.

Component	Desirable	Undesirable
Total cholesterol	less than 5.2 mmol/L (200 mg/dl)	5.2 mmol/L (200 mg/dl) or more
LDL	less than 3.36 mmol/L (130 mg/dl)	3.36 mmol/L (130 mg/dl) or more
HDL	more than 1.5 mmol/L (55mg/dl)	0.9 mmol/L (35 mg/dl) or less
Ratio of total cholesterol to HDL* less than 4.0		5.0 or more

[1] Total cholesterol level divided by HDL value.

Patients with Priorities for Testing

Being aware of our limited resources, the panel recommended that some Canadians be given priority over others in having all their blood lipids tested, at least initially. It also seemed hopeful that someday there would be enough laboratories and health care dollars to test all adult Canadians. This, however, brings us to cost effectiveness, something I fear we'll hear quite a bit more about in the future.

We forget how expensive lab tests can be because we don't pay for them directly; the bill is sent to our province's medicare program for payment. But in Ontario, for example, medicare has been paying almost $50 for a complete lipid screen. Were 10 million adult Canadians to be tested at that cost, the bill would approach $500 million. If each of those 10 million saw their doctors for a full physical examination first, that could cost another $500 million. Add to that those doctors' not unusual desire for tests of blood counts, sugars, liver function, thyroid function, and for such things as electrocardiograms and, with no trouble at all, the bill could hit $2 billion.

Then all the patients with elevated lipids would have the tests repeated at least once, perhaps twice. Some would be referred to specialists, hospitals, therapy programs and dietitians. They'd have follow-up exams with their doctors and those other health care professionals. Their blood tests would be repeated periodically to see how the diet and/or drug treatments were working. The final costs would be astronomical - even if there were enough professionals to take care of all those patients.

These are the costs of screening. Now to the benefits those costs must be balanced against. We'd need to calculate how many years, months or days of life our screening and other programs would save. Would those found to have elevated lipids live longer? Would they miss fewer days from work because they were diagnosed? When it comes to cost effectiveness, it's not enough to simply say that identifying those at risk would prevent coronary artery disease, heart attacks and deaths if they follow our advice.

If Canada had a surgeon-general, he or she would argue that there's absolute proof those with low cholesterols have significantly fewer heart attacks and heart-related deaths. He or she would pull out the numbers: for every 1 per cent drop in cholesterol over a period of years, there's a 2 per cent drop in the heart attack rate. Whatever the cost, routine screening for cholesterol is worth it.

An auditor-general would argue that even if heart attacks are prevented, people will still die - from cancer, accidents, suicide and a host of other causes. From the accounting point of view, a death is a death and screening for cholesterol doesn't necessarily save money. Auditor-generals look at statistics and dollars, not people.

Cost effectiveness analysis is far more complex than that, of course. There are all sorts of permutations and combinations to consider. But it is still a free country and that leaves me free to order the cholesterol and other blood tests I feel are necessary for my patients. It leaves you free to ask your doctor to order the tests if you'd like to have them. It leaves him or her free to refuse if you're a very healthy person with no other risk factors. But if at some point in the future provincial governments limit the number or type of blood tests doctors are allowed to order under medicare, we had all better hope we can still have the tests if we pay for them ourselves.

Governments have limited and will continue to limit what medicare plans will cover. It's a fact of life - we can't continue to spend endlessly on health care. Already some hospitals won't analyze for HDL unless the total cholesterol is elevated. This could be disastrous: you might have a normal total cholesterol with a very low HDL, putting you at high risk of a heart attack. And you wouldn't know until it was too late because fractionating the cholesterol into components was just too expensive for the hospital's budget.

Given this squeeze between health care and tax dollars, one of our brightest hopes is the Consensus Conference's recommendation for a push to make the public more aware of what preventive medicine has to offer. A concerted health promotion effort is required, and that will cost money. Not just the money we pay in taxes but also our donations to such voluntary agencies as the Heart and Stroke Foundation of Canada and the Canadian Atherosclerosis Society. If we can convince Canadians of the benefits of a low-fat, low-cholesterol diet and modification of other risk factors, perhaps we could then accept that only high-risk individuals need to have routine cholesterol screening.

Laboratory Services

There is no point in running blood tests if the results aren't reliable, and it's clear that some laboratories aren't performing these tests as well as they should. A 15 per cent error can turn a cholesterol of 6.0 into one of 5.1 mmol/L. At 6.0 you'd need treatment; if you were reported to be 5.1, you'd be neither diagnosed nor treated. In addition, as Chapter 3 outlines, some labs still consider you abnormal only if you have levels higher than 95 per cent of a population that is the same age and sex. Yet we know that being above the 75 per cent level just about doubles your risk of heart attack.

If you feel that these laboratories shouldn't be wasting our money this way, why not pressure your federal and provincial representatives to pay attention to the Consensus Conference recommendations.

Other Recommendations

What would I have added to the Consensus panel's final report? Well, for one thing, a recommendation that research on young people be started immediately. Quite apart from our concern that the young be as healthy as possible, we should remember it is their tax dollars that will be helping to support us in our old age - provided they don't start dying at 40 from heart disease. We need research on just how much fat those under 18 should be eating, whether 30 to 40 per cent of daily calories or 25 to 30 percent.

For another thing, I'd have mentioned that not only the general public needs better nutrition education, many doctors and some dietitians do, too. Another fact of life is that there's a lot of great-tasting high-fat food out there, and it's not likely to go away. Canadians enjoy eating it, and a whole segment of society depends on it for a livelihood. As a motivator, the carrot works better than the stick, and it's healthier for us, too.

No one ever had a heart attack because of the occasional hot dog or dish of gourmet ice cream. We have to teach everyone, including health care professionals, that life is not black or white; it's a far better place when you can see the greys. Rigid rules won't accomplish much, but some flexibility and humour may.

My tailor tells me that almost every one of his overweight clients claims to be dieting. Many ask if the suits they're ordering can be taken in after they lose weight. In all the years he's been in business, few have ever returned to be measured for a smaller size. And of those few, most had their suits let out again. "I've slipped back to my fatness wardrobe," they say. I know what they mean. I've been there myself, many times. And that's not the sort of flexibility I'm talking about.

Fat Content of Common Foods

This is a general guide to where the fats are in your food. It doesn't cover the fat content of every food, brand or cut of meat, but it does give you general counts for some of the key sources of dietary fat. Use this guide along with your knowledge of the different types of fat to learn more about what you're eating.

Once you've learned which foods have the most fat, you won't need to keep track of your daily intake. You'll automatically size up new food products, choose the lower-fat dishes in restaurants and cook low-fat meals at home.

| | Approximate Amounts of | | | | |
| | Fat | SFA | PUFA | Chol | Cal |
Milk and Milk Foods	*(g)*	*(g)*	*(g)*	*(mg)*	*(k)*
Milk, 8 oz. (250 mL), whole (homo)	9.0	5.0	tr.	35	159
2%	5.0	3.0	tr.	19	128
skim	0.3	tr.	tr.	5	90
Butter (see Fats and Oils)					
Cheese, 1-1/2 oz. (45 g). Read label to find percentage of fat, listed along with the letters B.F. (butterfat) or M.F. (milk fat)					
29 to 31% fat range (cheddar, gouda, gruyere, munster, swiss, parmesan, cream cheese, etc.) up to	15.0	9.0	tr.	47	181
around 15% fat (partly-skimmed mozzarella, ricotta, etc.)	7.0	5.0	tr.	27	118
7% fat range (low-fat and light cheeses such as skim milk slices and spreads)	3.0	2.0	tr.	16	86
Cottage cheese, 1/2 cup (125 mL), creamed 4.5% B.F.	5.0	3.5	tr.	17	119
2% B.F.	2.5	1.5	tr.	10	107
Cream, 1 tbsp. (15 mL) whipping, 35% B.F.	5.0	3.0	tr.	19	49
sour, 14% B.F.	2.0	1.0	tr.	6	23
coffee, 18% B.F.	3.0	2.0	tr.	9	28
half and half, 12% B.F.	2.0	1.0	tr.	6	20
Ice Cream, 1 cup (250 mL), gourmet type, 16% B.F.	24.0	6.0	tr.	92	368
regular, 10% B.F.	16.0	10.0	tr.	62	284
Sherbet, 1 cup (250 mL)	4.0	2.0	tr.	14	286
Yogurt, 125 g, frozen fruit, 6.3% B.F.	5.0	-	-	-	148
fruit flavour, 1.4% B.F.	2.0	1.0	tr.	7	131
plain, 1.5% B.F.	2.0	1.0	tr.	8	79

Meat, Poultry, Fish and Meat Substitutes

Because the fat values in this category can vary widely, we have in several cases given the averages for the many cuts and various types of cooking listed in *Nutrient Value of Some Common Foods*. Some days you may under-estimate the fat content from these foods; other days you'll over-estimate. It should average out over time. As Chapter 7 recommends, trim as much fat as you can, cook with little or no extra fat, and don't add batters or other coatings, sauces or gravies.

Meats	Fat (g)	*Approximate Amounts of* SFA (g)	PUFA (g)	Chol (mg)	Cal (k)
Beef, approx. 3 oz. (90 g)	12.0	4.9	tr.	65	213
Lamb, approx. 3 oz. (90 g)	12.0	6.8	tr.	84	204
Liver, approx. 3 oz. (90 g)	7.2	2.0	0.5	442	183
Pork, approx. 3 oz. (90 g)	12.0	4.0	1.2	59	209
Veal, approx. 3 oz. (90 g)	11.0	5.5	tr.	90	201

Deli or Luncheon-Type Meats

	Fat (g)	SFA (g)	PUFA (g)	Chol (mg)	Cal (k)
Blood sausage, 1 slice, 1 oz. (30 g)	10.0	4.0	1.0	36	113
Bologna, beef/pork, 1 slice, 3/4 oz. (23 g)	6.0	2.0	tr.	12	70
Ham, 1 slice cooked, 1 oz. (30 g)	3.0	tr.	tr.	15	49
Salami, beef/pork, 1 slice, 3/4 oz. (23 g)	4.0	2.0	tr.	14	55
Sausage, 1 beef/pork, 16 per 500 g pkge.	5.0	2.0	tr.	11	59
Wiener, 1 beef/pork, 12 per 450 g pkge.	11.0	4.0	1.0	19	118
Wiener, 1 turkey, 12 per 450 g pkge.	7.0	2.0	2.0	40	84

Poultry

	Fat (g)	SFA (g)	PUFA (g)	Chol (mg)	Cal (k)
Chicken, approx. 3 oz. (90 g)	5.8	1.4	1.2	72	157
Turkey, approx. 3 oz. (90 g)	4.5	1.0	1.0	66	148

Fish

	Fat (g)	SFA (g)	PUFA (g)	Chol (mg)	Cal (k)
Fatty (salmon, trout, mackerel, tuna, herring, sardines), approx. 3 oz. (90 g)	8.8	2.8	1.2	71	175
Lower-fat (cod, halibut, sole, whitefish, bluefish), approx. 3 oz. (90 g)	4.2	1.0	tr.	63	134
Shellfish (lobster, shrimp, scallops), approx. 3 oz. (90 g)	.7	tr.	tr.	87	97

Meat Substitutes

	Fat (g)	SFA (g)	PUFA (g)	Chol (mg)	Cal (k)
Egg, large, uncooked	6.0	2.0	tr.	274	79
Garbanzo beans or chick peas, cooked, 1 cup (250 mL)	4.0	tr.	2.0	0	284
Legumes (white beans, kidney beans, split peas), cooked 1 cup (250 mL)	1.0	tr.	tr.	0	238
Nuts (almonds, cashews, peanuts, pecans, pistachios, walnuts), 1/2 cup (125 mL)	36.0	4.5	10.3	0	403
Peanut Butter, 1 tbsp. (15 mL)	8.0	1.0	2.0	0	95
Seeds (pumpkin/squash, sesame, sunflower) 1/2 cup (125 mL)	38.0	5.3	19.6	0	431
Tofu, 1 piece (2-3/4 x 2-1/3 x 3/4 inch)	4.0	tr.	2.0	0	68

Fruits and Vegetables

All but a few fruits and vegetables are naturally fat-free. As long as you don't batter and fry them, or add overly fatty toppings, you can eat them to your heart's content. One exception is the avocado. While it contains mostly mono-unsaturated fats, don't lose sight of the fact that it's still a high-fat food - a Californian avocado (sold in winter) has 30 grams of fat; one from Florida (sold in summer and autumn) has 20 grams.

| | *Approximate Amounts of* | | | | |
| | *Fat* | *SFA* | *PUFA* | *Chol* | *Cal* |
Grains, Breads, Cereals and Pasta	*(g)*	*(g)*	*(g)*	*(mg)*	*(k)*
Bagel, 3-1/2 inches	2.0	tr.	tr.	0	200
Bread, tortilla, 1 piece	tr.	tr.	tr.	tr.	67
Hot dog or hamburger bun	3.0	tr.	tr.	3	164
Granola, homemade, 1/2 cup (125 mL)	17.0	3.0	9.0	0	312
Oatmeal, cooked, 1/2 cup (125 mL)	1.0	tr.	tr.	0	77
Noodles (canned chow mein type), 1 cup (250 mL)	11.0	tr.	tr.	5	230
Pasta (macaroni, spaghetti) cooked, 1 cup (250 mL)	1.0	tr.	tr.	0	164
Pasta (egg noodles), cooked, 1 cup (250 mL)	2.0	tr.	tr.	52	211
Barley, bulgar, 1/2 cup (125 mL)	1.0	tr.	tr.	0	349
Rice, brown, cooked, 1 cup (250 mL)	1.0	tr.	tr.	0	214

Most cold breakfast cereals have very little fat and usually no cholesterol, but the calorie count may be high if they're presweetened.

Baked Goods and Crackers

	Fat	SFA	PUFA	Chol	Cal
Cake, white layer with chocolate icing, 1/16th of 9-inch diameter	8.0	3.0	1.0	1	249
Cheesecake, 1/12th of 9-inch diameter	18.0	10.0	-	170	278
Cookies, 2, arrowroot	2.0	tr.	tr.	tr.	57
chocolate chip	5.0	1.0	1.0	9	104
peanut butter	7.0	2.0	1.0	11	123
Croissant, plain	12.0	4.0	1.0	13	235
Doughnut, plain, yeast-leavened	11.0	3.0	2.0	11	174
Fruit pie, two-crust, 1/16th of 9-inch diameter	18.0	5.0	4.0	0	412
Muffin, plain homemade type, medium-size	4.0	1.0	tr.	21	118

Crackers tend to be high in fat. Unless you know how much there is in your favourites, count each cracker (or two small thins) as having one gram of fat. Exceptions are melba toast, soda crackers, rice cakes and water biscuits for cheese, which you can count as being almost fat-free.

Snacks and Fast Foods	Fat (g)	SFA (g)	PUFA (g)	Chol (mg)	Cal (k)
English muffin, egg, cheese and bacon	18.0	8.0	tr.	213	360
Potato chips, small bag, 60 g	21.0	6.0	12.0	0	315
Popcorn, cooked in oil, no butter added, 1 cup (250 mL)	3.0	2.0	tr.	0	55
Pretzels, stick type, 5	tr.	tr.	tr.	0	59
Fish sandwich, large without cheese	27.0	6.0	10.0	91	470
Pizza, sausage, 1/4 of 14-inch	18.0	4.0	tr.	38	366
Hot dog, beef with bun	14.0	4.0	1.0	22	267
Taco with meat filling	11.0	4.0	tr.	21	195
Cheeseburger, 4 oz. patty	31.0	15.0	2.0	104	525
French fries, 10	8.0	3.0	tr.	7	158
Milkshake, thick chocolate, 1 cup (250 mL)	45.0	6.0	4.0	tr.	250
Hamburger, regular, 2 oz. patty	11.0	4.0	tr.	32	245
Roast beef sandwich	13.0	4.0	2.0	55	345

The typical chicken sandwich has 42 grams of fat; six chicken nuggets have about 13 g; and two pieces of fried chicken 25 g.

Fats and Oils

	Fat (g)	SFA (g)	PUFA (g)	Chol (mg)	Cal (k)
Butter, 1 tbsp. (15 mL)	11.0	7.0	tr.	31	100
Margarines, 1 tbsp. (15 mL)	11.0	2.0	3.5	0	100
Lard, 1 tbsp. (15 mL)	13.0	5.0	1.0	12	117
Shortening, 1 tbsp. (15 mL)	13.0	4.0	-	0	117
Oils, 1 tbsp. (15 mL), average for canola, corn, olive, peanut, soybean and sunflower (see Table 7.2)	14.0	2.0	6.0	0	124
Mayonnaise, over 65% oil, 1 tbsp. (15 mL)	11.0	1.0	4.0	8	102
Mayonnaise, over 35% oil, 1 tbsp. (15 mL)	5.0	2.0	2.0	4	58
Thousand Island commercial, 1 tbsp. (15 mL)	6.0	tr.	2.0	4	64
Blue cheese, 1 tbsp. (15 mL)	8.0	tr.	3.0	3	77
French, regular commercial, 1 tbsp. (15 mL)	6.0		tr.	2.0	9
64					
calorie-reduced, 1 tbsp. (15 mL)	2.0		tr.	tr.	tr.
24					
Homecooked, boiled, 1 tbsp. (15 mL)	2.0		tr.	tr.	9
25					

Dietary Fibre in Common Foods

It's generally agreed that soluble dietary fibre is particularly helpful in controlling cholesterol. The foods that are good sources of this are marked * on the following lists. But don't try to get just one type; choose a variety of fibre-rich foods, making sure you eat some of the soluble type each day. While fruits and vegetables can be fresh, dried, canned or frozen, you'll get more fibre if you can eat the skin. Juices have no fibre at all.

Because our bodies need time to adjust to higher-fibre foods, especially soluble sources like legumes, add extra amounts to your diet gradually and drink lots of liquids with them. Finally, don't be distracted by fancy names when buying crackers, cookies and cereals. Make sure you know what you're buying. The good old oatmeal cookie may have just as much fibre at half the price.

Whole Grain Foods	Fibre (g)	Approximate Amounts of SFA (g)	PUFA (g)	Chol. (mg)	Cal (k)
Rye bread, 1 slice dark, pumpernickel	1.0	tr.	tr.	tr.	79
Whole wheat bread, 1 slice 100%	1.4	tr.	tr.	tr.	61
Oatmeal, cooked, 1/2 cup (125 mL)	1.1	1.0	tr.	0	77
Brown rice, cooked, 1/2 cup (125 mL)	1.1	tr.	tr.	0	107
Bran muffin, home recipe, medium size	2.0	1.0	tr.	41	104
Spaghetti, enriched, cooked, 1 cup (250 mL)	1.2	tr.	tr.	0	164

Breakfast Cereals

	Fibre (g)	SFA (g)	PUFA (g)	Chol. (mg)	Cal (k)
Bran flakes, whole wheat, 3/4 cup (200 mL)	3.9	-	-	0	139
Bran, all bran, 1/2 cup (125 mL)	13.2	-	-	0	113
Bran, bran buds, 1/2 cup (125 mL)	10.7	-	-	0	122
Bran, 100%, 1/2 cup (125 mL)	9.9	tr.	tr.	0	90
Corn bran, 3/4 cup (200 mL)	6.1	-	-	0	118
Corn flakes, plain, 3/4 cup (200 mL)	tr.	-	-	0	70
Red River, cooked, 1/2 cup (125 mL)	2.4	-	-	0	82
Wheaties, 3/4 cup (200 mL)	1.7	tr.	tr.	0	86
Shreddies, 3/4 cup (200 mL)	3.2	-	-	-	169

Flour and Grains

	Fibre (g)	SFA (g)	PUFA (g)	Chol. (mg)	Cal (k)
Rye, flour, light, 1 cup (250 mL)	4.5	tr.	tr.	0	357
Wheat, flour, all purpose, 1 cup (250 mL)	3.9	tr.	tr.	0	484
Wheat, flour, whole, 1 cup (250 mL)	11.3	tr.	1	0	423

Fruits

	Fibre (g)	SFA (g)	PUFA (g)	Chol. (mg)	Cal (k)
*Apple, medium with skin	3.5	tr.	tr.	tr.	81
Apricots, dried, 5 halves, uncooked	1.4	tr.	tr.	0	41
fresh, 3 medium, raw	1.8	tr.	tr.	0	51
*Banana, medium	2.4	tr.	tr.	0	105
Blueberries, 1/2 cup (125 mL)	2.0	0	0	0	43
Cantaloupe, half	2.7	0	0	0	93
Cherries, 1 cup (250 mL)	1.8	tr.	tr.	0	110
Dates, pitted, chopped, 1/2 cup (125 mL)	7.2	0	0	0	258
*Grapefruit, half, pink	1.6	tr.	tr.	0	37
*Orange, medium, raw, peeled	2.6	tr.	tr.	0	62
Peach, medium, raw, no skin	1.2	tr.	tr.	0	37
*Pear, canned halves, juice packed, 1 cup (250 mL)	4.8	tr.	tr.	0	131
medium, raw, with skin	4.7	tr.	tr.	0	100

	Fibre (g)	Approximate Amounts of			
Whole Grain Foods		SFA (g)	PUFA (g)	Chol. (mg)	Cal (k)
Pineapple, 1 cup (250 mL) raw, diced	2.3	tr.	tr.	0	80
Plum, raw, medium size	1.1	tr.	tr.	0	36
*Prunes, dried, uncooked, 10	10.0	tr.	tr.	0	201
Raisins, seedless, 1 cup (250 mL)	15.1	tr.	tr.	0	522
Raspberries, frozen, sweetened,					
1 cup (250 mL)	13.5	tr.	tr.	0	272
Raspberries, raw, 1 cup (250 mL)	6.6	tr.	tr.	0	64
*Strawberries, frozen, sweetened, whole,					
1 cup (250 mL)	5.4	tr.	tr.	0	210

Vegetables

Asparagus, cooked, 1/2 cup (125 mL)	1.4	tr.	tr.	0	48
Bean sprouts, mung, cooked, 1/2 cup (125 mL)	0.7	tr.	tr.	0	14
*Beans, green , cooked, 1/2 cup (125 mL)	1.7	tr.	tr.	0	23
*Broccoli, cooked, 1/2 cup (125 mL)	2.3	tr.	tr.	0	24
Brussels sprouts, cooked, 1/2 cup (125 mL)	2.5	tr.	tr.	0	32
*Cabbage, cooked, 1/2 cup (125 mL)	1.6	tr.	tr.	0	17
*Carrots, cooked, 1/2 cup (125 mL)	2.5	tr.	tr.	0	37
*Cauliflower, cooked, 1/2 cup (125 mL)	1.1	tr.	tr.	0	16
Celery, raw, diced, 1/2 cup (125 mL)	1.0	tr.	tr.	0	10
*Corn kernels, cooked, 1/2 cup (125 mL)	2.4	tr.	tr.	0	70
Parsnips, cooked, 1/2 cup (125 mL)	2.9	tr.	tr.	0	67
Peas, green cooked, 1/2 cup (125 mL)	3.8	tr.	tr.	0	71
*Potato, medium, peeled before boiling	1.4	tr.	tr.	0	116
large, baked in skin, flesh and skin	3.5	tr.	tr.	0	163
Spinach, cooked, 1/2 cup (125 mL)	2.2	tr.	tr.	0	22
raw, chopped, 1 cup (250 mL)	2.4	tr.	tr.	0	13
*Sweet potatoes, cooked without skin,					
1/2 cup (125 mL)	4.2	tr.	tr.	0	182
Tomato, medium	1.8	tr.	tr.	0	23
Turnip, cooked, 1/2 cup (125 mL)	2.6	tr.	tr.	0	22

Legumes

*Kidney beans, cooked, 1/2 cup (125 mL)	3.3	tr.	tr.	0	119
*Lima beans, cooked, 1/2 cup (125 mL)	4.7	tr.	tr.	0	111
*Lentils, cooked, 1/2 cup (125 mL)	4.2	tr.	tr.	0	122
*Peas, cooked, 1/2 cup (125 mL)	2.4	tr.	tr.	0	122
*Navy beans, cooked, 1/2 cup (125 mL)	4.1	tr.	tr.	0	132

*Good source of soluble fibre

A 30-Gram Fibre Day

You may find it difficult to imagine what a high-fibre diet will be like. It's not really that unusual, as this sample menu shows.

Breakfast	*Grams of Fibre*
Cooked oat bran cereal (3/4 cup)	3.5
Small handful raisins (about 1/4 cup)	3.0
Skim milk (1/2 cup)	0.0

Mid-morning snack

Bran muffin or medium banana	2.5

Lunch

Salmon sandwich filling	0.0
Whole wheat bread (2 slices)	4.8
Split pea soup (about 1/2 cup peas)	4.7
Skim milk (1 cup)	0.0
Orange for dessert	2.5

Dinner

Poached chicken breast	0.0
Baked potato and skin	2.5
Mixed broccoli and carrots (1 cup)	5.0
Small green salad (estimate)	1.0
Skim milk (1 cup)	0.0
Strawberries (1 cup)	3.0

Total fibre for the day	32.5

A Look at Some of the Science

You've likely noticed throughout this book references to less than ideal experimental methodologies and to questionable interpretations of some studies and their results. Indeed, virtually every study that has been done has come under some critical scrutiny. Without question, the medical community is divided on how to interpret study results and how much of an effort should be made to perform screening blood cholesterol measures on people at low risk of heart disease. Then there is controversy about when and if drug treatment should be initiated.

Since I think the relationship between blood cholesterol and coronary artery disease is an important one, before you read some examples of what I feel is less than ideal science, I'd better explain why I've taken the stand that I have. There is no question in my mind that many studies actually do not prove what they have purported to prove. As well, I don't believe that some official recommendations, particularly those in other countries, are justified based on today's knowledge. We had better be very careful in exposing individuals to drug therapy, unless their blood cholesterols are dangerously high and all non-drug therapies have failed.

However, in my opinion, there is every logical reason for the entire population to adopt a prudent diet. Enough circumstantial evidence exists to strongly support the recommendation to reduce fat intake in general and to limit saturated fats to 10 per cent of calories. No evidence exists that I am aware of to suggest that this recommendation will in any way harm people. Thus the potential benefits in reduced heart disease, and possibly cancer, without doubt outweigh any potential deleterious effects. Likewise, increasing the amount of complex carbohydrate and fibre in the diet while reducing total protein, and specifically animal-derived protein, seems totally logical. Again, the potential benefits are many; the detriments none, that we know of.

To reject a prudent diet and other risk-factor modification based on the notion that there have been no studies that prove statistical significance, just does not make sense. Not when there is every indication that a prudent diet is far healthier than the diet most Canadians now consume.

One common argument made against many of the intervention studies is that although the incidence of heart-related problems including death decreased, the actual death rate did not. In other words, treating people for their elevated cholesterol did not prevent death, it just changed the cause of death. That should not surprise anyone. We are all mortal.

In one of the major studies, the deaths prevented by lowering blood cholesterols were lost owing to an increased rate of suicide and homicide. Some might interpret this to mean that taking the drug involved somehow promotes violent death. Or they might say why treat elevated cholesterols when no lives were saved. Those of us not interested in dying of heart attacks can see the fallacy of such an interpretation.

An analysis of current data by some researchers revealed that for low-risk middle-aged people, a lifelong cholesterol lowering program would add something between three days and three months to their lives. For people at high risk, the benefits of extra life would be in the range of 18 days to 12 months. Actually, when you consider the time spent in doctors' offices, waiting rooms and with nutrition counsellors, the benefits might well be reduced to minutes of extra life. What you have to remember, however, is that these are statistical analyses. You and I are flesh and blood, not numbers.

The recommendations in this book are based on those of the Canadian Consensus Conference on Cholesterol, and on my review of the literature. They are, in my opinion, reasonable and logical. They are intended to identify people at increased risk of heart disease and to modify that risk. They are not a panacea guaranteeing immortality.

I present the following study information so that you will understand why it would be unprofessional to adopt some of the recommendations of other bodies that exceed the Canadian Consensus recommendations.

WHY LIMITING EGGS AND OTHER HIGH CHOLESTEROL FOODS
MAY NOT BE NECESSARY

My wife makes a luscious dish called Seafood in Love. It's a combination of shrimps, scallops, lobster and a Hollandaise-type sauce. What a combination from a cholesterol point of view: seafood, egg yolks and butter! Although we usually replace the butter with Becel, the margarine that contains the largest percentage of polyunsaturates (see Chapter 7), Seafood in Love is still swimming in an ocean of dietary cholesterol. The question is, will adhering to a prudent diet mean no more Seafood in Love?

Does a prudent diet mean no more omelettes? No more eggs at all? Is the current recommendation for a diet containing 300 mg or less of cholesterol per day scientifically sound?

My answer to all those questions is, "It depends on the person." My wife and I will continue to have Seafood in Love, not every night but perhaps a couple of times a year. That's all we ever had it anyway. After almost 18 years of marriage there's only so much love, with seafood, a person can take.

As far as cholesterol intake goes, eggs are a relatively inexpensive source of protein. If I like them and I'm not allergic, I should feel free to eat them. Let's delve into why I feel that way.

A large uncooked egg has 274 mg of cholesterol. Eat just one and, if you were trying to keep your intake under 300 mg, the remainder of your day's food would have to be vegetarian. If you added a cup of whole milk with 33 mg of cholesterol or an ounce of cheddar with 30 mg, you'd be over 300 for the day. Just one single boiled egg for breakfast and three ounces of sirloin steak for dinner would give you a daily total of 341 mg. Add three ounces of canned salmon for lunch and you'd be hitting 378.

One egg plus 3-1/2 ounces of boiled shrimp equal 469 mg of dietary cholesterol. But few people eat only a single egg. Most omelettes call for two eggs; he-men have omelettes with three eggs in them. And everyone knows that shrimps eaten by themselves need to be dipped in garlic butter for maximum enjoyment. A mere tablespoon of butter has 31 mg of cholesterol.

However, my problem with the 300 mg daily limit is based not on a love of shrimp with lots of garlic butter but on the fact that I can find little justification for it in the medical literature.

How are Cholesterol Studies Done?

Like much of the research on nutrition, studies dealing with the relationship between dietary and blood cholesterol are done in one of several ways: on animals with the results being extrapolated to people; on people who do not represent the general public; on very small numbers of people; on people sequestered in a hospital's metabolic ward; on people not eating normal diets; on people fed diets containing ludicrous amounts of cholesterol; or on sick people.

The consensus of all the studies, regardless of the merits of their scientific methods, is this:

1. For much of the population, the amount of cholesterol in the diet has little or nothing to do with blood cholesterol, HDL or LDL.

2. Of all dietary factors, such as fat, saturated fat and polyunsaturated fat, the cholesterol content of food has the least influence on blood cholesterol levels.

That's the reason for the change of heart about seafood. Once, those who had elevated cholesterol or were simply watching their levels were advised to cut shrimp and other fatty seafood from their diets. Then came the new word: seafood fatty acids are excellent. For most people, the cholesterol in seafood does not affect blood levels one way or another.

You'll notice that there is a qualification to all this. *Not everyone reacts the same way.* The levels in perhaps a third of the population (I don't think anyone knows for sure) will increase if they are fed a diet high in food containing cholesterol. What seems evident from reviewing the literature is that there is no sure-fire way to predict who these people are. They may have high, low or average cholesterol levels. They may have healthy or unhealthy arteries. They may have normal LDLs and HDLs. They may be overweight or underweight.

About the only way to identify these "hyper-responders" is to try various diets. I'm not aware of anyone doing a study on this, but the medical literature really has no other suggestions I could understand. Let us review, then, a couple of studies from respected medical journals.

Two Cholesterol Studies

In the *British Medical Journal*, February 7, 1987, research dietitians and scientists at the Radcliffe Infirmary, Oxford, published the results of their study on subjects fed reduced-fat, high-fibre diets. Healthy volunteers were recruited through newspaper advertisements; of 194 applicants, 35 were rejected because they weren't as healthy as they thought and 24 others were excluded later because they felt unable to stick to the diet. If my subtraction is correct, that left Radcliffe with results from 135 participants. Interestingly, 108 of them were women. In most other studies on lipids, the majority of the subjects are men. Could it be that healthy men are not as likely to volunteer for such a study? Were many of the 24 who withdrew men? (One can always ask questions about study methods.)

In addition to the 135 healthy people, 20 men and 13 women with elevated serum lipids were included in the 24-week study. During the first eight weeks, all 168 were asked to follow an individualized low-fat, high-fibre diet. The number of calories varied from 1,000 to 3,000 a day, depending on how many each person required to maintain stable body weight. However, the most commonly prescribed diet contained 1,500 calories. I find that a bit strange, since the recommended daily number for a middle-aged woman is 1,800 to 2,000. A deficit of 300 to 500 calories a day, 2,100 to 3,500 a week, should cause the loss of up to a pound a week, even though the study's aim was to keep body weights constant.

The 1,500-calorie diet prescribed for the healthy people had 15 per cent of its calories as protein, 50 per cent as carbohydrate and 35 per cent as fat. The polyunsaturated/saturated fat ratio was 0.6. (The prudent diet's recommendation is about 1.0.) The 1,500-calorie diet prescribed for those with elevated lipids was slightly different: 18 per cent protein, 56 per cent carbohydrate and 26 per cent fat, with a P/S ratio of 0.8.

For the first eight weeks, participants were asked to get used to their diets - all of which were to include *two* eggs per week. Then they were divided into two groups and, for the next eight weeks, one group continued with the same diet; the other increased its egg intake to *seven* per week. So that saturated fat and calorie levels would remain constant, some minor changes were made to their diets to compensate for the five eggs' extra protein and fat.

A Cross-Over Study

During the last eight weeks, the group that had been eating two eggs per week was asked to eat seven. And the group that had been eating seven was cut back to two. This is what is called a "cross-over study." After a run-in period of eight weeks to get everyone established on the low-fat diet, the design allows the researchers to compare people with themselves (how they did on two vs. seven eggs per week) and with everyone else. This allows one to look at individual as well as group trends.

The average age of the 168 participants was 45 years; the average body mass index was 24.8 when the study began and 23.9 after the run-in period. That should be no surprise, as we predicted a weight loss. However, during the next 16 weeks of the experiment, the body weights didn't change. I am not sure how to explain that. The participants apparently kept records of what they ate and followed the diets given them. As another check of compliance, the fatty acid compositions of their triglycerides were measured. Those who adhered to the diets should have showed a sustained increase in linoleic acid (a polyunsaturate), since the low-fat diets were formulated that way.

What Were the Results?

The healthy group had an average "initial pretreatment" cholesterol of 5.45 mmol/L. I assume that represents their average cholesterol after the run-in period. After four weeks of eating two eggs per week, the average fell to 5.17 mmol/L; after eight weeks at two eggs per week, it was 5.23. At seven eggs per week, the corresponding numbers were 5.32 after four weeks and 5.33 after eight. There is a statistically significant difference between the four-week values of 5.17 and 5.32, but not between the eight-week values of 5.23 and 5.33.

In other words, after eight weeks there was no difference in the cholesterol levels of the healthy people who ate two or seven eggs per week. There was no difference in the levels of those eating 350 mg of cholesterol per day and those eating 150 mg per day.

The small difference at four weeks was not seen in the group that had high blood lipids to begin with. Whether its members ate seven eggs per week or two, whether their average daily cholesterol intake was 308 mg or 120, there was no effect on their blood cholesterol levels at any time.

Why the Study Was Done

The national average egg intake in Britain is four per week. This study was intended to see whether halving or almost doubling that average had any effect on cholesterol in otherwise healthy people or in those who had elevated cholesterols. We could fault the study on the grounds that the healthy group was put on a diet with a fat content of 35 per cent rather than the recommended 30 per cent, and received a higher than recommended proportion of saturated fat as well. But on the whole, it does what it intended to do, using normal, active people who were not put into a hospital and fed artificial diets. There were also more women that men in the sample for a change. This could be important because virtually everything that associates blood cholesterol with coronary artery disease involves studies predominantly composed of middle-aged men.

Note that the study doesn't tell us what happens if dietary cholesterol in healthy people goes above 350 mg per day, or what effect dietary cholesterol has on those with lower P/S ratios (eating diets higher in saturated fats). It doesn't identify the group that other researchers claim is very sensitive - those hyper-responders who have marked increases in their cholesterol levels when dietary cholesterol is increased. Perhaps they weren't identified because this study lasted for weeks instead of days, allowing everyone's system to adjust to the diets.

What the study does tell us is that for those attempting to keep their saturated fat levels low (P/S ratios high), eating up to seven eggs per week or 350 mg of cholesterol per day is not likely over time to raise blood cholesterol. It does not support a recommendation suggesting that dietary cholesterol be restricted to 300 mg per day. Nor does it suggest that eating more than 350 mg per day is safe.

How Does the Body Control Cholesterol?

Before we look at another study and its results, a review of how the body controls its cholesterol levels is important. You'll remember that cholesterol is not an essential nutrient; our livers are capable of producing all our bodies require. Even if we ate no cholesterol at all, we shouldn't become deficient. What factors then, could possibly control our cholesterol levels? We don't yet know for certain - any of the following may have something to do with the process:

1. The amount of cholesterol our livers produce.
2. The amount our intestines absorb from food.
3. The amount our bodies process or use as building blocks in cells and to produce various hormones.
4. The amount our body is able to store. The more we store out of the blood, the lower our cholesterol levels will be.
5. The amount we can excrete from our bodies.

One of the prerequisites of life is that animal cells need a relatively constant environment. Human beings are no exception. We control the temperature around us by our choice of clothing, with various forms of shelter, with air conditioners and heaters. Our bodies control our chemical compositions with far greater precision. Our potassium levels, for instance, range from 3.5 to 5.0 mmol/L. Anything more or less and we might well be in life-threatening trouble. Considering all the other mechanisms and fluid compositions the body has to keep constant, it only stands to reason that some system exists to regulate our cholesterol.

What might happen is that when we increase the amount of cholesterol in our diets, our liver compensates by producing less or we excrete more in the stool. The net result would be to keep the blood cholesterol at a more or less constant level. It may take a bit of time for these compensatory mechanisms to kick in, and perhaps the study just reviewed demonstrates this time lag. After four weeks of two eggs per week, blood cholesterols were lower than after four weeks of seven eggs per week. By eight weeks, however, levels were equal whether on two or seven eggs. It may have taken the bodies of the participants more than four but less than eight weeks to compensate for the cholesterol in five extra eggs per week.

A Study of Middle-Aged Men

An American study, published in the *Journal of Clinical Investigation*, Volume 79, June 1987, looks at some of the body's mechanisms to determine how we react to changes in the type of fat we eat and the quantity of cholesterol in our diets. The scientists were from The Rockefeller University in New York.

In their introduction, the researchers list 20 other studies showing that people fed cholesterol reacted by decreasing the amount their livers made and/or by excreting more in the stool. Their bodies reacted to the increased amount in food by shutting down internal cholesterol production and eliminating extra cholesterol, with the net effect of keeping blood levels relatively constant. In one study mentioned, there was evidence to suggest that when faced with increased amounts of cholesterol in the diet, some people absorb less. So decreased absorption from food may be another way of lowering elevated cholesterol levels. Other people may produce and excrete extra bile as another mechanism to eliminate cholesterol from the body, while others may store excess cholesterol in various body cells.

Fifty middle-aged men were used in this study and, while we're not told specifically, the implication is that they had elevated cholesterol levels. None had symptoms of heart disease. Each received dietary counselling and was taught how to assess the size of food portions. Divided into two groups, designated SFA and PUFA, each had a diet in which 35 per cent of calories came from fat. However, the SFA group had a high saturated-fat diet (P/S 0.3) while the PUFAs had a high polyunsaturated fat diet (P/S 1.5).

During the first six weeks of the study, both groups ate relatively little cholesterol. Then each man was asked to eat three large eggs per day for the next six weeks. (An unbroken string of he-man omelettes, perhaps?) To compensate for the extra protein and calories, an appropriate amount of meat/fish/poultry was deleted from their diets. Finally, 25 of the 50 changed from SFA to PUFA, 25 from PUFA to SFA, and they began the study all over again.

The researchers checked blood samples and diet diaries at various times during the study. With recently developed technology, they were able to analyze changes in the body's production of cholesterol and the absorption of cholesterol from food. Throughout the low-cholesterol part of the study, the average participant ate about 240 mg of cholesterol per day; when the three large eggs were added, he was consuming about 840.

And the Results Were . . .

On average, the amount of cholesterol the men absorbed from their food decreased. And so did the amount of cholesterol produced in their bodies. As expected, those in the high-PUFA group had lower average cholesterol levels than the group on the high saturated-fat diet. However, going from about 240 to 840 mg of dietary cholesterol a day didn't seem to alter average levels in either group. Nor were HDL levels affected by the change from a low- to high-cholesterol diet.

There were some patients who *did* respond with significant increases in their cholesterol levels. According to the report, eight of 75 fell into this category. Since there were supposedly only 50 participants, I don't know how to calculate the percentage these eight represent. Interestingly, though, the levels of three men went the opposite way. With increasing levels of dietary cholesterol, their blood levels fell significantly.

The authors concluded that dietary cholesterol content had marginal influence on lipid levels in the blood. Based on this, they rejected the recommendation that the entire population needs to lower intake from the current average level of about 450 mg per day to less than 300 mg. However, they did find in their study a group that was sensitive to increased dietary cholesterol. For these hyper-responders, the amount in the diet may well be very important. Unfortunately, there is no way to determine who they are, other than to test them using different diets.

HOW SOME OF THE GOOD FAT, BAD FAT
STUDIES WERE DONE

Roughly 40 per cent of the calories consumed by the average North American come from fat. Nearly all experts consider a diet with more than 35 per cent coming from fat, a high-fat diet. Therefore, most North Americans are consuming a high-fat diet.

But as we all know by now, there is fat, and there is fat. To put it in the simplest terms, there is good fat, there is neutral fat, and there is bad fat. Have you ever wondered how this is decided?

In many studies where researchers tried to look at groups of people in order to establish a relationship between diet and atherosclerosis, the researchers concluded that the more fat people eat, the more likely they are to develop heart disease. Some of the studies divided the fats eaten into their components, and these studies have tended to show that there is a relationship between the amount of saturated fat that people eat, their blood cholesterol levels, and coronary artery disease.

It has become clear, however, that life is more complicated than that. The notion that all saturated fats are bad, that mono-unsaturated fats are neutral, and that all polyunsaturated fats are good, simply doesn't stand up to scientific scrutiny. The idea that people who want to prevent heart disease must avoid all red meat, seafood and eggs, is just not true.

Much of the research that has been done related specific fatty acids to increased or decreased levels of blood cholesterol, and this conclusion leaves much to be desired. A good deal of the research was supported by special interest groups, such as a segment of the fat and oil industry, a marketing board or a lobby group of some sort. Let's take a look at some of this research.

A Study from Texas

Doctors Andrea Bonanome and Scott Grundy, of the Center for Human Nutrition, University of Texas Southwestern Medical Center at Dallas, published an article in the May 12, 1988 issue of the much-quoted *New England Journal of Medicine.* Their study was meant to determine if stearic acid raises blood cholesterol levels. Stearic acid is a completely saturated, fatty acid whose main dietary sources are beef and cocoa butter.

As to the study method, 11 men were chosen to take part in this study. We're not told how they were chosen. Four had a history of coronary heart disease and throughout the study took calcium-channel blockers, beta-blocking drugs, and nitroglycerine. Presumably, the other seven men were healthy and taking no medication during the study.

How would these 11 men measure up to a randomly chosen group of 11 men from your neighbourhood or mine? Their average age was 64; average weight 72 kg; average body mass index (BMI) 24. On those facts, I'd say these 11 men were older than the average person in my medical practice, my neighbourhood, and the city I live in. (And notice that no women were included in the study sample.) We can't tell much from the men's average weight because we're not told their average height. The average BMI tells us that they might be a tad over "ideal" weight.

In general, these men were part of the group that requires at least a prudent diet if they want to get their blood serum cholesterol level down to the magic 5.2. I calculated that their average cholesterol:HDL ratio was 5.29, which puts them at greater than average risk of heart attack. This should not surprise us, considering average age and the fact that four were under treatment for coronary artery disease. We're not told how many times the men's lipid levels were measured before the study began.

Now to consider the actual study. This study was divided into three periods lasting three weeks each. During those nine weeks, the men were fed liquid formula diets in which 40 per cent of the calories came from fat, 40 per cent from glucose (simple sugar, not complex carbohydrates), and 20 per cent from milk proteins. The men's cholesterol intake was less than 100 mg per day. During the whole study period, the men were confined to the metabolic ward of the Dallas Veteran's Administration Medical Center. They were allowed to walk around the hospital grounds, but they were forbidden to take any strenuous exercise.

Flaws in the Study Method

Sorry to be giving you all these details, but anyone who wants to evaluate the results of a study has to be sure that he or she thinks the method chosen by the researchers was adequate to answer the questions posed, and that it supports the researchers' conclusions. In this instance - and, unfortunately, this is the rule with these sorts of studies - you needn't have a PhD in research design to see the flaws.

For starters, these 11 men weren't typical of the population in general. Other than the facts that four of them had heart disease and that all were older than average, we don't know much about them. Next, you and I and most other members of our communities are not confined to the metabolic ward of a hospital. Just being in an institution, regardless of diet, would alter such things as our blood pressures, our mental states, and our blood lipids. Nor do you and I live on liquid diets. And even when we did, as infants, it's to be hoped that 40 per cent of our calories didn't come from pure glucose.

Although I'm an MD and have a master of science degree, I'm still not a professional expert on study design. Even so, the circumstances have so far not impressed me with the methodology used in this study.

Now, of course, we'll want to know what fats were used in the men's diets during the three phases of the study period. One diet was high in palmitic acid, a saturated fatty acid. In this diet, palm oil was the only source of fat.

Another diet was high in stearic acid, the fatty acid that the researchers actually wanted to study. You'll remember my saying that dietary sources of stearic acid were beef and cocoa butter? Well, maybe they had trouble getting stearic acid in natural form - they had a synthetic fat made by Anderson Clayton Foods, courtesy of the W.L. Clayton Research Center of Richardson, Texas.

To make this synthetic fat, the processors took a mainly polyun-saturated soybean oil and completely hydrogenated it. They then took their now-saturated product and chemically hydrolyzed and randomly re-esterified it with safflower oil, and "the resulting product was prepared as the fat" for the 11 men's liquid diet.

I am not a chemist. But I have to wonder what all the hydrogen-ating, hydrolyzing, and re-esterifying did to the soybean and safflower oil. The final mixture contained some mono-unsatu-rates, polyunsaturates, and saturates other than stearic acid. How many of them exist in nature?

Let's not lose sight of the study protocol. The researchers were trying to find out whether stearic acid, presumably as it's found in my diet and yours, causes blood cholesterol levels to go up, go down or stay the same. Considering the methodology described, do you think this study was well enough designed to find the answer?

The third diet had a fat component high in oleic acid, a mono-unsaturated fatty acid. For this diet, they say, a high oleic-contain-ing safflower oil was used. It sure must have been an unusual safflower oil because the percentage of oleic acid given is far higher than that of the safflower oil I know. Perhaps they made a clerical error, or maybe the safflower oil had its fatty acids modified with a little hydrogenation, giving it trans-bonds and other unnatural things.

The Results Seemed Promising

Now that we know the method, we can consider the results. None of the 11 men died. Just as surprising, none of them dropped out of the study. Only very highly motivated men would stay cooped up in a veterans' hospital for nine weeks, drinking those luscious diets. They drank their meals, maintained their weight, and reported no adverse effects. The results:

- The men's average blood cholesterol level was 14 per cent lower on the stearic acid diet than it was on the palmitic acid diet. Their LDL was 22 per cent lower. Their HDL was not affected.
- Their average blood cholesterol was 10 per cent lower on the oleic acid diet than it was on the palmitic diet. Their LDL was 15 per cent lower. Their HDL was not affected.
- Their average blood cholesterol, LDL and HDL were about the same when they were on the oleic acid and stearic acid diets.

The authors discussed the results of their study, of course. Customarily, this section of a scientific publication begins with a review of the literature written earlier on the subject. These authors did not break with custom. They cited seven studies previously published, all of which concluded that stearic acid did not raise blood cholesterol. Yet, they said, few people seem to have taken much heed of this. As a result, stearic acid continued to be lumped with the other saturated fatty acids, and so people continued to assume that eating foods containing it would elevate their cholesterol.

Were the Comparisons Valid?

The researchers went on to suggest that the earlier studies were actually intended to examine other fatty acids that were more abundant in a normal human diet. Their study, however, was specifically designed to look at stearic acid. That's why they had an artificial fat made to produce a 42.9 per cent stearic acid content. Nature doesn't offer any food that has a content approaching 45 per cent and they wanted to compare stearic acid with palmitic acid. The source of the latter they chose was palm oil, which contains 43 to 45 per cent palmitic acid. Yet they compared these two diets with a third that they said contained 79.7 per cent oleic acid. Why didn't they pick a third fatty acid that had from 40 to 45 per cent to make the comparisons valid?

When the men were on the stearic acid diet, their average total cholesterol dropped to 4.47 mmol/L from 5.87; while they were on the oleic acid diet, it dropped to 4.68. The figures suggest that the diet containing the artificial fat with all those saturates lowered their cholesterol more than a diet rich in polyunsaturates. We can only guess what fats these men were consuming before the study, because when they were on the palmitic acid diet - which had a total saturated fat content of 51.1 per cent mmol/L - the average level fell to 5.22 mmol/L from 5.87.

It seems that no matter what they fed these 11 men, their cholesterol levels fell. Could something other than the fat component of the diets account for these results?

Certain Limitations

The reason the total cholesterols of all 11 dropped, said the researchers, was that the men had been on even poorer diets before the study began. Likely they were consuming more cholesterol. But they also noted the curious outcome that people's blood cholesterol levels tend to fall when they go into the metabolic ward of a hospital. The researchers couldn't explain why this might happen, yet it does.

In the end, they did recognize "certain limitations" in their study. It couldn't really be used to come to any conclusion about what stearic acid does to women. And since the men in the study were kept on special diets, the researchers "urge that the results not be extended unreservedly to common fats rich in stearic acid, such as beef fat and cocoa butter, without further evidence" to support the results. This is especially important, they pointed out, because beef fat and cocoa butter also contain palmitic acid, which they say "was clearly shown to raise the cholesterol [level]" - even though their study showed that it actually lowered it.

Their conclusion was that all saturated fats are not the same in their effects on blood cholesterol. This conclusion, they said, must be taken into account when the experts make their recommendations. They suggested that foods containing stearic acid be developed - for example, a margarine containing stearic acid would provide texture without raising cholesterol. That was their final remark. And that's the one that will stick in the minds of most people.

An Editorial and an Interview

Also in the May 12, 1988 edition of the *New England Journal of Medicine* was an editorial by Doctors I.H. Rosenberg and E.J.

Schaefer of the USDA Human Nutrition Research Center on Aging, at Tufts University. It reminded us that all the studies referenced by the researchers were carried out while the subjects were on liquid formula diets that contained about 40 per cent fat and less than 100 mg of cholesterol. "It is likely," they concluded, "that the finding with high-stearic-acid diets would apply to non-formula diets with a higher cholesterol content, but this remains to be verified." I would have thought it far safer to conclude that it's of no use to speculate on this finding until further studies are completed.

In addition, they mentioned that the food industry would be interested to know that margarines high in stearic acid may be as useful as those high in linoleic acid for reducing blood cholesterol. At the same time, such margarines may have a nicer texture and a better taste.

Dr. Grundy, one of the authors of the stearic acid study, was interviewed in the May 27, 1988 issue of a journal called *Science*. In the interview he said the study showed that "lean beef is okay. It has an acceptable role in our diet." He also believed that by using stearic acid in the processed food industry, it would be possible to create a more palatable diet, while still keeping cholesterol levels down.

Mark Hegsted, identified as a Professor Emeritus at Harvard University, was interviewed for the same report in *Science*. He was reported to have said: "Stearic acid does not raise cholesterol, but I don't believe it lowers cholesterol. It lowers cholesterol [as] compared to palmitic acid. But [that] doesn't mean the more stearic acid you eat, the lower your cholesterol will go."

Back to Grundy: "It is a plus for beef. It turns out [that] beef raises cholesterol less than we thought." How this conclusion was reached on the basis of his study of liquid diets and the caveat published is beyond me. Remember the caveat? The researchers urged "that the results not be extended unreservedly to common fats rich in stearic acid, such as beef fat and cocoa butter, without further evidence." Perhaps some evidence came to light between the time that statement appeared in the *New England Journal of Medicine* on May 12 and the time the *Science* interview was published on May 27.

Remember, too, that his study was done on 11 aging men, none of whom were allowed to eat beef. Heck, they were barely allowed to go for a walk. Interviews like this tend to make a person doubtful, to say the least.

Conclusions are Difficult

Talking in general terms about a subject as complex as this leaves us open to future criticism. On the other hand, it's difficult to be specific in a field where we still have a tremendous amount to learn about the specifics.

In this book I've done my best to make recommendations based on today's knowledge. I hope, though, that in the very near future there will be an explosion of knowledge about lipids and about preventing heart disease. Properly conducted studies may find that some of today's recommendations were off-base. But until that happens, I recommend that you follow the dictum "moderation in all foods" - except, of course, for the complex carbohydrates.

Index

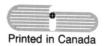

Printed in Canada